T0362551

On-the-Field Emergencies

Editors

ERIC MCCARTY
SOURAV PODDAR
ALEX EBINGER

CLINICS IN SPORTS MEDICINE

www.sportsmed.theclinics.com

Consulting Editor
MARK D. MILLER

July 2023 • Volume 42 • Number 3

ELSEVIER

1600 John F. Kennedy Boulevard ● Suite 1800 ● Philadelphia, Pennsylvania, 19103-2899

http://www.theclinics.com

CLINICS IN SPORTS MEDICINE Volume 42, Number 3
July 2023 ISSN 0278-5919, ISBN-13: 978-0-443-18191-7

Editor: Megan Ashdown
Developmental Editor: Malvika Shah

Clinics in Sports Medicine (ISSN 0278-5919) is published quarterly by Elsevier Inc., 360 Park Avenue South, New York, NY 10010-1710. Months of issue are January, April, July, and October. Business and Editorial Offices: 1600 John F. Kennedy Blvd., Ste. 1800, Philadelphia, PA 19103-2899. Customer Service Office: 3251 Riverport Lane, Maryland Heights, MO 63043. Periodicals postage paid at New York, NY and additional mailing offices. Subscription prices are $379.00 per year (US individuals), $773.00 per year (US institutions), $100.00 per year (US students), $421.00 per year (Canadian individuals), $953.00 per year (Canadian institutions), $100.00 (Canadian students), $494.00 per year (foreign individuals), $953.00 per year (foreign institutions), and $235.00 per year (foreign students). Foreign air speed delivery is included in all *Clinics* subscription prices. All prices are subject to change without notice. **POSTMASTER:** Send address changes to *Clinics in Sports Medicine*, Elsevier Health Sciences Division, Subscription Customer Service, 3251 Riverport Lane, Maryland Heights, MO 63043. Customer Service (orders, claims, online, change of address): Elsevier Health Sciences Division, Subscription Customer Service, 3251 Riverport Lane, Maryland Heights, MO 63043. **Tel: 1-800-654-2452 (U.S. and Canada); 314-447-8871 (outside U.S. and Canada). Fax: 314-447-8029. E-mail: journalscustomerservice-usa@elsevier.com (for print support); journalsonlinesupport-usa@elsevier.com (for online support).**

Reprints. For copies of 100 or more of articles in this publication, please contact the Commercial Reprints Department, Elsevier Inc., 360 Park Avenue South, New York, NY 10010-1710. Tel.: 212-633-3874; Fax: 212-633-3820; E-mail: reprints@elsevier.com.

Clinics in Sports Medicine is covered in *MEDLINE/PubMed (Index Medicus) Current Contents/Clinical Medicine, Excerpta Medica,* and *ISI/Biomed.*

Contributors

CONSULTING EDITOR

MARK D. MILLER, MD
S. Ward Casscells Professor, Head, Department of Orthopaedic Surgery, Division of Sports Medicine, University of Virginia, Charlottesville, Virginia; Team Physician, Miller Review Course, Harrisonburg, Virginia

EDITORS

ERIC MCCARTY, MD
Professor, Chief of Sports Medicine and Shoulder Surgery, Department of Orthopedics, University of Colorado School of Medicine, Head Team Physician, University of Colorado, Sports Medicine and Performance Center, Boulder, Colorado

SOURAV K. PODDAR, MD
Associate Professor, Team Physician, University of Colorado, Sports Medicine–Colorado Center, Denver, Colorado; Associate Professor, Departments of Family Medicine and Orthopedics, University of Colorado School of Medicine, Aurora, Colorado

ALEX EBINGER, MD
Assistant Professor, University of Colorado, Associate Professor, Department of Emergency Medicine, University of Colorado School of Medicine, Aurora, Colorado

AUTHORS

BARRY P. BODEN, MD
Sports Medicine, University of Georgia, Athens, Georgia

RON COURSON, ATC, PT, SCS, NRAEMT, CSCS
Executive Associate Athletic Director, Sports Medicine, University of Georgia, Athens, Georgia

WILLIAM DENQ, MD, CAQ-SM
University of Arizona, Tucson, Arizona

ALEX EBINGER, MD
Assistant Professor, University of Colorado, Associate Professor, Department of Emergency Medicine, University of Colorado School of Medicine, Aurora, Colorado

KATLYN ELLIOT, MD
Family Medicine Resident, McKeesport Family Medicine Residency, University of Pittsburgh Medical Center, McKeesport, Pittsburgh

JIM ELLIS, MD
Sports Medicine, University of Georgia, Athens, Georgia

GHASSAN FARAH, MD
Department of Orthopaedic Surgery, University of Illinois, Chicago, Illinois

OMAR FARAH, BS
Columbia University Vagelos College of Physicians and Surgeons

JEFFREY P. FEDEN, MD, FACEP, FAMSSM
Associate Professor, Clinician Educator, Department of Emergency Medicine, The Warren Alpert Medical School of Brown University, Providence, Rhode Island

RACHEL M. FRANK, MD
UCHealth CU Sports Medicine - Colorado Center, Denver, Colorado

ALECIA GENDE, DO, CAQSM
Assistant Professor of Orthopedics, Departments of Emergency Medicine and Sports Medicine, Mayo Clinic Health System, La Crosse, Wisconsin

GEORGIA GRIFFIN, MD
Sports Medicine Fellow, University of Washington Sports Medicine Center, Department of Family Medicine, Section of Sports Medicine, University of Washington, Seattle Children's Hospital, Seattle, Washington

GLENN HENRY, MA, PMDC
Sports Medicine, University of Georgia, Athens, Georgia

CHRISTOPHER P. HOGREFE, MD, FACEP, CAQ-SM
Clinical Associate Professor, Department of Emergency Medicine, University of Iowa Hospitals and Clinics, University of Iowa Carver College of Medicine, Iowa City, Iowa; Adjunct Associate Professor, Department of Orthopaedic Surgery, Northwestern Medicine, Northwestern University Feinberg School of Medicine, Chicago, Illinois

MARK R. HUTCHINSON, MD
Distinguished Professor of Orthopaedic Surgery and Sports Medicine, Department of Orthopaedic Surgery, University of Illinois, Chicago, Illinois

CALVIN ERIC HWANG, MD
Clinical Assistant Professor, Department of Orthopaedic Surgery, Stanford University School of Medicine, Stanford, California

MICHAEL IBRAHEM, MD
Family Medicine Resident, Shadyside Family Medicine Residency, University of Pittsburgh Medical Center, Pittsburgh, Pittsburgh

RYAN A. KEENAN, MD
Primary Care Sports Medicine Fellow, University of Colorado School of Medicine, University of Colorado, Aurora, Colorado

OLIVIA KELLER-BARUCH, MD
Emergency Medicine Resident, University of Missouri, Columbia, Missouri

ROSS E. MATHIASEN, MD, CAQ-SM
Associate Professor, Department of Emergency Medicine, University of Nebraska Medical Center, Omaha, Nebraska

ERIC MCCARTY, MD
Professor, Chief of Sports Medicine and Shoulder Surgery, Department of Orthopedics, University of Colorado School of Medicine, Head Team Physician, University of Colorado, Sports Medicine and Performance Center, Boulder, Colorado

SALMA MUMUNI, MD
Department of Orthopaedic Surgery, University of Illinois, Chicago, Illinois

MATTHEW NEGAARD, MD, CAQ-SM
Assistant Professor, Department of Emergency Medicine, University of Iowa, Iowa City, Iowa; Sports Medicine Physician, Forte Sports Medicine and Orthopedics, Indianapolis, Indiana

BEN OSHLAG, MD, CAQ-SM
White Plains Hospital, White Plains, New York

SOURAV K. PODDAR, MD
Associate Professor, Team Physician, University of Colorado, Sports Medicine–Colorado Center, Denver, Colorado; Associate Professor, Departments of Family Medicine and Orthopedics, University of Colorado School of Medicine, Aurora, Colorado

STEVEN K. POON, CASQM, MD
Instructor in Orthopaedics, Senior Associate Consultant, Sports Medicine Section, Department of Orthopaedic Surgery, Mayo Clinic, Phoenix, Arizona

ASHWIN L. RAO, MD
Professor, Department of Family Medicine, Section of Sports Medicine, University of Washington, University of Washington Sports Medicine Center, Seattle, Washington

ROBB REHBERG, PhD, ATC, NREMT
Sports Medicine, University of Georgia, Athens, Georgia

HEATHER ROESLY, MD, CAQSM
Emergency Medicine Faculty, University of Colorado, Aurora, Colorado; UC Health Highlands Ranch Hospital, Highlands Ranch, Colorado

KARTIK SIDHAR, MD
Clinical Assistant Professor, Department of Family Medicine, University of Michigan Medical School, Ann Arbor, Michigan

LEINA'ALA SONG, MD
Sports Medicine Fellow, University of Washington Sports Medicine Center, Department of Family Medicine, Section of Sports Medicine, University of Washington, Seattle, Washington

JAMES P. STANNARD, MD
Chief Medical Officer for Procedural Services, Hansjörg Wyss Distinguished Chair in Orthopaedic Surgery, Chairman, Department of Orthopaedic Surgery, Medical Director, Missouri Orthopaedic Institute, University of Missouri, Columbia, Missouri

JAMES T. STANNARD, MD, PhD
Department of Orthopaedic Surgery, University of Missouri, Columbia, Missouri

DANIEL J. STOKES
UCHealth CU Sports Medicine - Colorado Center, Denver, Colorado

ALEXANDER J. TOMESCH, MD, CAQ-SM
Assistant Professor, Department of Emergency Medicine, University of Missouri, Columbia, Missouri

JESSICA TSAO, MD, MSc
Clinical Instructor, Department of Medicine, Stanford University School of Medicine, Stanford, California

JENS T. VERHEY, MD
Resident in Orthopaedics, Department of Orthopaedic Surgery, Mayo Clinic, Phoenix, Arizona

ELAN VOLCHENKO, MD
Department of Orthopaedic Surgery, University of Illinois, Chicago

MARY TERESE WHIPPLE, MD
Assistant Professor, Departments of Emergency Medicine, and Orthopedics and Rehabilitation, University of Iowa Hospitals and Clinics, Iowa City, Iowa

Contents

The foundation of preventing and treating an on-field emergency is preparation and readiness. The sideline medical team should coordinate the utilization of an emergency action plan (EAP). A successful EAP is accomplished through attention to detail, rehearsal, and self-assessments. Every EAP should include site-specific implementation, personnel, equipment, communication, transportation, venue location, emergency care facilities, and documentation. Improvements and advancements can be made to the EAP by self-evaluation after each on-field emergency and yearly reviews. A competent sideline emergency medical team can enjoy the competition while being ready to respond to a catastrophic on-field emergency.

The collapsed athlete encompasses multiple critical and noncritical pathologic conditions, management of which highly depends on the elements of presentation of an athlete, the environment in which the athlete presents, and the key history elements leading to the collapse. Early identification of an unresponsive/pulseless athlete with basic life support/CPR, AED use, and EMS activation is key, with the addition of early hemorrhage control in acute traumatic injuries. The initiation of a focused history and physical examination is critical to rule out life-threatening causes of collapse and to guide initial management and disposition.

Cardiac-related deaths are the leading nontraumatic cause of death in the young athlete. Although there are multiple causes for cardiac arrest in athletes, sideline evaluation and management does not vary. Recognition, immediate high-quality chest compressions, and time to defibrillation are the greatest factors affecting survival. This article reviews the approach to the collapsed athlete, causes for select cardiac emergencies in athletes, preparedness for cardiac emergencies, and return to play considerations and recommendations.

Emergent airway issues are rare in competitive sports. However, when airway compromise occurs, the sideline physician will be relied upon to manage the situation and the airway. . The sideline physician is tasked with not only the evaluation of the airway, but also management until the athlete can get to a higher level of care. Familiarity with the assessment of the airway and the various techniques for the management of airway compromise on the sideline are of the utmost importance in the unlikely event that an airway emergency should occur.

Injuries to the chest and thorax are rare, but when they occur, they can be life-threatening. It is important to have a high index of suspicion to be able to make these diagnoses when evaluating a patient with a chest injury. Often, sideline management is limited and immediate transport to a hospital is indicated.

Acute hemorrhage in sport is a common issue for the sideline professional. The severity of bleeding ranges from mild to severe and life- or limb-threatening. The mainstay of management of acute hemorrhage is achieving hemostasis. Hemostasis is frequently accomplished via direct pressure but may require more invasive management including tourniquet use or pharmacologic management. With concerns for internal bleeding, dangerous mechanism of injury, or signs of shock, prompt activation of the emergency action plan is required.

The presentation of traumatic abdominopelvic injuries in sport can range from initially benign appearing to hemorrhagic shock. A high clinical suspicion for injury, knowledge of the red flags for emergent further evaluation, and familiarity with the initial stabilization procedures are necessary for sideline medical providers. The most important traumatic abdominopelvic topics are covered in this article. In addition, the authors outline the evaluation, management, and return-to-play considerations for the most common abdominopelvic injuries, including liver and splenic lacerations, renal contusions, rectus sheath hematomas, and several others.

This article focuses on the management of the most common on-field medical emergencies. As with any discipline in medicine, a well-defined plan and systematic approach is the cornerstone of quality health care delivery. In addition, the team-based collaboration is necessary for the safety of the athlete and the success of the treatment plan.

discuss appropriate treatment at the athletic venue. Fractures that can be seen with athletic activities include cervical spine; knee osteochondral fractures; tibia, ankle, and clavicle. Dislocations that will be considered include knee, patella, hip, shoulder, sternoclavicular joint, and proximal interphalangeal joint of the finger. These injuries vary significantly both in severity and in the emergent nature of the injury.

Acute Compartment Syndrome in the Athlete

Omar Farah, Ghassan Farah, Salma Mumuni, Elan Volchenko, and Mark R. Hutchinson

In sports, acute compartment syndrome (ACS) develops following lower limb fracture, with subsequent high intracompartmental pressures and pain out of proportion to the physical examination. A prompt diagnosis is the key to a successful outcome in patients with ACS. The goal of treatment of ACS, namely decompressive fasciotomy, is to reduce intracompartmental pressure and facilitate reperfusion of ischemic tissue before onset of necrosis. A delay in diagnosis and treatment may result in devastating complications, including permanent sensory and motor deficits, contractures, infection, systemic organ failure, limb amputation, and death.

CLINICS IN SPORTS MEDICINE

THE CLINICS ARE AVAILABLE ONLINE!
Access your subscription at:
www.theclinics.com

CLINICS IN SPORTS MEDICINE

Foreword

Hours of Boredom, Punctuated by Moments of Sheer Terror

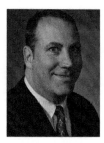

Mark D. Miller, MD
Consulting Editor

It is unclear exactly who gets credit for this quote, but it has been used to describe warfare, flying, poker, playing outfield in baseball, anesthesiology, and…team coverage. This phrase came to mind when I was covering a gymnastics event at a local university several years ago. Our program was devoid of both scholarships and talent, and we were competing against some of the better teams in our region. Needless to say, I was nervous every time one of our gymnasts ran down the ramp to the pommel horse, and there were plenty of "miss-mounts." The one thing that can reduce the risk of sheer terror in this arena is something we can borrow from the Boy Scout Motto: Be Prepared!

The timing of this issue of *Clinics in Sports Medicine* couldn't have been better. But, I must admit that it was sheer luck that we planned this issue well before the Damar Hamlin incident brought this topic into the national spotlight. Fortunately, the medical teams covering that infamous Bills versus Bengals NFL game were prepared and literally saved this young man's life. It is essential that EMTs, Athletic Trainers, Team Physicians, and anyone covering athletics be ready for any catastrophic event that may occur in an otherwise mundane, or even boring, competition. This requires vigilance to stay current on diagnosis and treatment of on-field emergencies, maintaining credentials, and practice. We can help with the first requirement—just read this treatise!

Thank you to the tremendous medical team at the University of Colorado—Home of Coach Prime Time. Drs McCarty, Poddar, and Ebinger put together a fantastic issue that covers everything from sudden collapse to traumatic injuries. These three team physicians come from different specialties and bring amazing insight to those of us that cover sports. As a member of the Presidential line of the American Orthopaedic Society for Sports Medicine (AOSSM), I would be remiss if I didn't put in a plug for what our society has planned to help you manage on-the-field emergencies. Look for a new Phone App and a new Master's Team Physician course to be announced

Clin Sports Med 42 (2023) xiii–xiv
https://doi.org/10.1016/j.csm.2023.03.002
0278-5919/23/© 2023 Published by Elsevier Inc.

soon. Because, as our motto notes—"We keep you in the game" (and help you prepare for moments of sheer terror).

Mark D. Miller, MD
Division of Sports Medicine
Department of Orthopaedic Surgery
UVA Orthopaedic Center at Ivy Road
2280 Ivy Road
Charlottesville, VA 22903, USA

E-mail address:
MDM3P@hscmail.mcc.virginia.edu

Preface

On-the-Field Emergencies in Athletics: It Takes a Team!

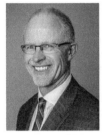
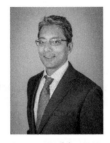
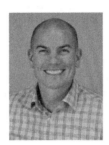

Eric McCarty, MD   Sourav Poddar, MD   Alex Ebinger, MD

Editors

Sports medicine is an ever-evolving field, with the focus on maintaining the health and well-being of athletes, both on and off the field. Most of the time, the sports medicine practitioner watches an event as a spectator available for occasional consultation for the athlete for a myriad of musculoskeletal injuries or for medical problems requiring treatment and determination of return to play. However, infrequently, there are times that the sports medicine practitioner is faced with emergent issues that can be as serious as life or death.

The topic of on-field emergencies has been brought to the forefront of national attention with the 2023 NFL Monday night football game in which Buffalo Bills safety, Damar Hamlin, collapsed on the field in cardiac arrest. The quick response and actions of the physicians, athletic trainers, and paramedics were paramount in saving his life. Most of the time the sports medicine clinician will not be faced with this type of scenario, yet it may happen, and one must prepare for this as well as for a multitude of other on-the-field emergencies.

In this issue of *Clinics in Sports Medicine*, we have been challenged by Dr Mark Miller to bring forth a collaborative, multidisciplinary approach to on-the-field emergencies. As guest editors, we represent three distinct, yet intertwined specialties: orthopedic surgery, family medicine, and emergency medicine. We work athletic events together and represent the multidisciplinary approach fostered in sports medicine at the University of Colorado, and thus, it was easy for us to collaborate in putting forth this issue.

Clin Sports Med 42 (2023) xv–xvii
https://doi.org/10.1016/j.csm.2023.03.003
0278-5919/23/© 2023 Published by Elsevier Inc.

We have brought together experts from various medical fields, including athletic trainers, orthopedic surgeons, family medicine physicians, emergency medicine physicians, general surgeons, and subspecialty physicians and surgeons, to provide a comprehensive review of the important aspects of on-field emergencies in athletics. Our aim is to provide a comprehensive and up-to-date overview of this critical area, exploring the latest research, best practices, and key considerations for managing these potentially catastrophic events. Whether you are a seasoned sports medicine practitioner or new to the field, this issue provides valuable insights and practical advice to enhance your ability to manage on-the-field emergencies with confidence and competence.

The articles of this *Clinics in Sports Medicine* issue are broad and inclusive, covering topics such as preparation and readiness for on-field sports emergencies and general principles of approaching the collapsed athlete. Following that, the articles will then become more focused on life-threatening emergency issues, such as cardiac arrest, which will be addressed in the article on Cardiac Emergency in the Athlete. Other topics with potentially fatal outcomes are covered by dual-trained emergency and sports medicine physicians, in articles devoted to the following: Acute Emergency Airway Issues in Sports, Chest/Thorax Injury in the Athlete, Acute Bleeding on the Playing Field, and Emergency Abdominopelvic injuries. Other articles covered by dual-trained family medicine and sports medicine specialists include the topics of General Medical Emergencies in Athletes, Heat and Cold and Other Environmental Emergencies in the Athlete, Emergency Facial Injuries in Athletics, and the ever-evolving Management of the Head Injury Emergency. The latter part of this issue includes an excellent multidisciplinary article on the Acute and Emergent Spinal Injury Assessment and Treatment. Last, renowned orthopedic team physicians have written articles on Management of Emergent Fractures and Dislocations on the Playing Field, and the Management of the Acute Compartment Syndrome in the Athlete.

We applaud Dr Miller, who for over two decades has provided the vision and leadership in editing the *Clinics in Sports Medicine*. He suggested this very relevant topic before it garnered national attention with the Hamlin scenario. Over 30 years have passed since this topic was covered in the *Clinics in Sports Medicine* series, thus it is overdue and particularly useful. We are thankful to all the experts from across the country who volunteered their time and devoted their expertise in writing outstanding articles. Last, we are thankful for each other, our families, and the wonderful profession that we have in sports medicine, which is rewarding and particularly enjoyable when you work with great people.

We hope that this *Clinics in Sports Medicine* issue will provide valuable insights and information for athletic trainers, team physicians, and emergency personnel, who are on the front line in responding to on-field emergencies. This issue is a must-read for all those involved in sports medicine, and we are confident that it will serve as a valuable resource for years to come.

Eric McCarty, MD
University of Colorado Champions Center
2150 stadium drive
Boulder, CO 80309, USA

Sourav Poddar, MD
University of Colorado
Sports Medicine–Colorado Center
Denver, CO 80222, USA

Alex Ebinger, MD
University of Colorado
Anschutz Medical Campus
Aurora, CO 80045, USA

E-mail addresses:
eric.mccarty@cuanschutz.edu (E. McCarty)
sourav.poddar@cuanschutz.edu (S. Poddar)
alexander.ebinger@cuanschutz.edu (A. Ebinger)

On-Field Sports Emergencies
Preparation and Readiness

Timothy P. McCarthy, MD[a],*, Rachel M. Frank, MD[b],
Daniel J. Stokes, MD[b], Eric McCarty, MD[a]

KEYWORDS

- On-field emergency • Emergency action plan • Sports medicine team
- Emergency training

KEY POINTS

- Preventative medicine through preparticipation physical evaluations plays a critical role in screening for conditions that may be life-threatening or predispose to injury or illness.
- An emergency action plan (EAP) is fundamental for a medical team to prepare and respond to an emergency and prevent catastrophic fatalities.
- There is a legal basis for developing and applying an EAP, and the absence of one has been the basis for negligence claims and lawsuits.
- EAP preseason training allows the team to practice various on-field scenarios and develop cohesion in preparation for athletic events throughout the season.
- Preparation and readiness for on-field emergencies are accomplished through attention to detail, self-assessments, leadership, and communication. A well-educated and devoted medical team and sufficient rehearsal ensure sideline emergency response competency.

INTRODUCTION

Athletics are a cornerstone of "culture" worldwide, with continued growth and participation during the last 2 decades. In 2019, nearly 8 million adolescents participated in school-related sporting activities, according to the 2018 to 2019 High School Athletics Participation Survey conducted by the National Federation of State High School Associations (NFHS).[1] Athletic participation at the youth, high school, collegiate, and professional level have an inherent risk for injury. Although most injuries in athletics are relatively minor, limb-threatening or life-threatening injuries are often unpredictable and can occur without warning. From 2011 to 2014, the Centers for Disease Control and Prevention reported nearly 5.6 million injuries related to sports or recreation

[a] CU Sports Medicine and Performance Center, Department of Orthopedic Surgery, 2150 Stadium Drive, Boulder, CO 80309, USA; [b] UCHealth CU Sports Medicine - Colorado Center, ATTN, 2000 South Colorado Boulevard, Tower 1, Suite 4500, Denver, CO 80222, USA
* Corresponding author. Department of Orthopedic Surgery, CU Sports Medicine and Performance Center, 2150 Stadium Drive, Boulder, CO 80309
E-mail address: Timothy.McCarthy@cuanschutz.edu

Clin Sports Med 42 (2023) 335–344
https://doi.org/10.1016/j.csm.2023.02.001
0278-5919/23/© 2023 Elsevier Inc. All rights reserved.

among persons aged 5 to 24 years.[2] Most of these injuries were not limb-threatening or life-threatening. However, during the 2017 to 2018 academic year in high school and collegiate athletes, there were 99 catastrophic injuries. A catastrophic injury is defined as fatalities, permanent disability injuries, temporary or transient paralysis, heat stroke due to exercise, sudden cardiac arrest, severe cardiac disruption, or serious injuries (cervical spine or head injuries) where the athlete made a full recovery.

Team medical coverage has evolved rapidly and has become a pivotal component of athletics at all levels of competition. The ultimate responsibility for medical decisions regarding prevention and treatment rests with the athletic health-care team, including the medical director, team physicians, athletic trainers, and allied health-care providers. Although the athletic health-care team has multiple roles and responsibilities, the core goal is preventing injury and managing on-field emergencies. Professional organizations have published guidelines on emergency preparedness, and state high school athletic associations have issued policies based on those professional guidelines. The National Athletic Trainer's Association (NATA) has published a position statement outlining the 12 best practice guidelines for athletic organizations (**Table 1**).[3]

There is broad agreement that the most effective way to prevent catastrophic fatalities and manage nonfatal catastrophic events is through a sound and well-rehearsed emergency action plan (EAP).[4] The EAP is the foundation for the medical team to prepare and respond to an emergency and should be readily available to all athletics and emergency medical system community members. It should be located centrally at each venue where athletic activities will occur.

NEED FOR EMERGENCY ACTION PLAN

Emergencies are never predictable but when they occur, a swift and coordinated response is the difference between effective and ineffective management. Government entities, including the military, law enforcement, and fire rescue, have established emergency plans to intervene in an emergency scenario. Athletes have an inherent risk of an emergency requiring timely access to emergency medical services (EMS). Given this risk, there is an organizational and professional responsibility for an EAP to be in place.

The National Collegiate Athletic Association (NCAA) has recommended that all institutions develop an emergency plan for their athletic programs.[5] The NFHS has echoed this recommendation at a high school level.[6] Despite these recommendations, there has been variable adoption and implementation of EAPs. At the high school level, 55% to 100% adoption with only 9.9% compliance with the guidelines recommended by the NATA.[7] In a questionnaire-based study of high schools across the United States, 70% of trainers reported that their schools had a written emergency response plan. Still, only 26% of the schools practiced the EAP throughout the year, and 36% never practiced.[8]

Along with organizational and professional responsibility, there is a legal basis for developing and applying an EAP. Sports medicine programs require well-formulated, adequately written, and periodically rehearsed emergency response protocols. The absence of an EAP has been the basis for claims and lawsuits based on negligence.[9]

PREPARING FOR THE SEASON
Preseason Physicals

The idea of preventative medicine plays a critical role in the setting of organized athletics. Before the start of a season, preparticipation physical evaluations (PPE) are

Table 1
National Athletic Trainer's Association position statement: best practice recommendations

1	Each institution or organization that sponsors athletic activities must have a written emergency plan. The emergency plan should be comprehensive and practical yet flexible enough to adapt to any emergency
2	Emergency plans must be written documents and distributed to certified athletic trainers, team and attending physicians, athletic training students, institutional and organizational safety personnel, institutional and organizational administrators, and coaches. The emergency plan should be developed in consultation with local emergency medical services personnel
3	An emergency plan for athletics identifies the personnel involved in carrying out the emergency plan and outlines the qualifications of those executing the plan. Sports medicine professionals, officials, and coaches should be trained in automatic external defibrillation, cardiopulmonary resuscitation, first aid, and prevention of disease transmission
4	The emergency plan should specify the equipment needed to carry out the tasks required in an emergency. In addition, the emergency plan should outline the location of the emergency equipment. Further, the equipment available should be appropriate to the level of training of the personnel involved
5	The establishment of a clear mechanism for communication to appropriate emergency care service providers and identifying the mode of transportation for the injured participant are critical elements of an emergency plan
6	The emergency plan should be specific to the activity venue. Each activity site should have a defined emergency plan derived from the overall institutional or organizational policies on emergency planning
7	Emergency plans should incorporate the emergency care facilities to which the injured individual will be taken. Emergency receiving facilities should be notified in advance of scheduled events and contests. Personnel from the emergency receiving facilities should be included in developing the emergency plan for the institution or organization
8	The emergency plan specifies the necessary documentation supporting the implementation and evaluation of the emergency plan. This documentation should identify responsibility for documenting actions taken during the emergency, evaluation of the emergency response, and institutional personnel training
9	The emergency plan should be reviewed and rehearsed annually, although more frequent review and rehearsal may be necessary. The results of these reviews and rehearsals should be documented and indicate whether the emergency plan was modified, with further documentation reflecting how the plan was changed
10	All personnel involved with the organization and sponsorship of athletic activities share a professional responsibility to provide for the emergency care of an injured person, including developing and implementing an emergency plan
11	All personnel involved with the organization and sponsorship of athletic activities share a legal duty to develop, implement, and evaluate an emergency plan for all sponsored athletic activities
12	The administration and legal counsel of the sponsoring organization or institution should review the emergency plan

important at all competition levels. In 2019, the American Academy of Pediatrics published updated PPE guidelines. The general goal of the PPE is determining general physical and psychological health and evaluating for life-threatening or disabling conditions, including the risk of sudden cardiac arrest and other conditions that may predispose the athlete to illness or injury.[10] It may also provide an entry point into the health-care system for those who do not otherwise have an established primary care physician. The primary objectives are to screen for conditions that may be life-threatening or disabling, conditions that may predispose to injury or illness, and to meet administrative requirements. The evaluation should include examining the cardiovascular, musculoskeletal, and neurologic systems. Additional screening for mental health, including depression, anxiety, and attention-deficit/hyperactivity, is also recommended.[10]

REVIEW OF POLICIES AND PROCEDURES

Before hosting athletic events, every institution must formulate an EAP, which should be developed and reviewed annually as a coordinated effort by the medical team, school administrators, local EMS, and first responders.[11] The EAP should undergo review at the beginning of each season. This review ensures that the protocols and policies are in place for the medical care of the athletes. This should occur at all levels of competition, and the personnel involved will be based on the level of the organization. At the high school level, this includes a conversation with the high school athletic trainer and athletic director before the school year and before the season. At a collegiate level, a review and update of the written policies and discussion with the athletic training staff includes a review of the NCAA published sports medicine handbook. At a professional level, written policies from the league and a team discussion with the head athletic trainer and management are reviewed.

PRESEASON ON-FIELD EMERGENCY TRAINING

Before the start of each season, time is dedicated to preseason training focused on preparing for the rigors of the upcoming training. This training allows the team to practice on the field and develop cohesion as a group. It will enable focused time for the team to establish the core principles and to practice various scenarios during competition throughout the season. The preseason training is the foundation on which success is based during the season. This foundation is then built on and fine-tuned throughout the season for continued improvement.

For the athletic health-care team, similar preseason training is vital to establish a foundation for success during the season. This preseason training should be a dedicated time for which all health-care team members should be present, including physicians, athletic trainers, EMS, and any other members involved. This should be repeated before the beginning of each new season. It provides a chance to review the EAP for that organization. It can also allow new members and veterans to work together and understand their roles during the season.

The most important aspect of preseason training is the rehearsal of various emergent scenarios that may occur throughout the season. This is a low-stress, hands-on opportunity for team members to practice the EAP for many on-field scenarios. Variations are associated with caring for an athlete on various surfaces, including grass, turf, court, or ice. Practicing at the appropriate venue distinguishes these variances. When preparing for a downed athlete, practicing spine boarding in multiple positions, including supine, prone, against a wall, or on the bench, will allow the team to be ready for any situation. This training also provides a chance to discuss and understand the medical and playing equipment, such as helmets, shoulder pads, or other protective gear.

Preparation will pay great dividends for providing care to an athlete in a live scenario. In these moments, it is easy to crack under pressure considering all eyes of teams, players, officials, and the crowd are on the athletic health-care team. Practice will provide the foundation for perfect execution when the pressure is on.

GAME DAY POLICIES AND PROCEDURES
Implementation

Once an EAP is written, it must be distributed to all medical personnel for familiarization and training. The emergency plan should be a brief schematic that is easy to understand. This allows a rapid, synchronous response from all medical team members.[12] A quick reference visual representation in a flowsheet or diagram is often the most practical.

Each member of the medical response team should familiarize themselves with the EAP. Educational sessions should be conducted to specify venue-specific nuances, including mapping the location of emergency equipment and communication devices. Education should also establish medical coverage qualifications, emergency equipment handling, and a communication approach to contact the local medical facility. A copy of the emergency plan should be located on the sideline in a designated location and made aware to all team members. Additionally, each member should receive a personal copy of the emergency plan with clearly defined roles.[4]

Implementation is only complete with practice. The medical team should practice emergency response situations. A well-designed emergency plan with many rehearsals resolves minor hitches, leading to an efficient and effective response in a setting that would otherwise incite panic and disorder. Successful implementation of an EAP is achieved through an easy-to-follow written plan, a thoroughly educated team, and a rehearsed response.

Personnel

A copy of the EAP should be distributed to all medical personnel, including the team physician, consulting physicians/residents, athletic trainers/students, coaches, and any other member of the sports medicine team. The EAP should demonstrate the qualifications of the primary medical team implementing the plan in emergent situations.[13]

Depending on the level of competition, the medical personnel may vary. As the competition level increases, the medical team typically increases as well. Although a high school game often only requires one physician, it may be unobtainable for a single physician to meet the needs of a collegiate or professional organization. High-level competition typically consists of multiple physicians, consultants, subspecialists, and athletic trainers. With increased personnel, it is critical to define roles and set expectations for each team member.

A chain of command can establish a structured approach to avoid uncertainty and confusion. The team physician can utilize this method to simplify and optimize productivity and communication with the team. Similar to any successful athletic organization, the medical team must work as a cohesive unit for peak performance. The lead physician should meet with all personnel before an event with expectations and responsibilities. Defining roles provides clarity and creates accountability. It also limits concern for a member taking on too much responsibility.[12,14]

As the medical team leader, the head physician must develop rapport with the athletes, coaches, and families. This can be achieved simply by being present and available to the athletes. Developing relationships enhances trust and decreases anxiety in emergent situations allowing the medical personnel to perform optimally. This may ultimately be the difference in life-threatening circumstances.

More recently, there has been an emphasis on the head physician and medical staff exercising independent medical judgment with management and return-to-play decisions for players. This is an advancement in limiting the discernment of conflict of interest between organizations and the welfare of a player. The increased responsibility of the medical team for health-care decision-making further reveals the importance of a team effort.[15] A well-prepared and compatible team, through defined roles and chain of command, can operate in a time-sensitive manner and potentially avert a major disaster.

Equipment

Emergent situations can sometimes require medical equipment. The EAP should include any equipment needed for an on-field emergency. Equipment should only be operated by trained medical personnel.

Although the goal is to avoid using emergency equipment, there are situations where it may be lifesaving. This equipment should be readily available at the venue and in operating condition. Routine checks should be performed to confirm that all equipment is functional and ready for use. All staff and medical personnel should be briefed on where to find this equipment. Creating maps with this information is beneficial, especially if this equipment is not immediately available on the sidelines.

Understanding how to use the equipment is imperative. With continuous advancements in medical technology, it is essential to maintain training for proper application and utilization. A member of the sideline medical team should be proficient in automated external defibrillator, oxygen, and advanced airways.

The American Heart Association has described a chain of survival critical response model that implements early recognition and activation of the emergency response team to perform cardiopulmonary resuscitation (CPR) and early defibrillation. The probability of survival is drastically increased with immediate CPR and defibrillation administered within 3 minutes.[16] Additional advanced life support measures include emergency oxygen supplementation and establishing an advanced airway through intubation.[17] A trained medical team with knowledge of the equipment and the ability to execute the EAP can increase survival.[18]

Communication

A critical requirement in any emergent response is communication. The EAP should establish communication guidelines and protocols for establishing transportation to an emergency care facility. The sideline medical team needs access to a telephone or other communication devices, including a list of emergency contacts and their locations.

As with the equipment, routine checks should be made to guarantee functional communication devices. Communication checks should be completed before each practice and game. Still, technology is not guaranteed, and a backup plan should be conceived.

Meeting the opposing medical team before a game to discuss logistics can be advantageous. This provides an overview of the available medical personnel, venue layout, and confirmation of communication and equipment location.[19] These fundamental communication tactics can help accelerate an emergency response and prevent dire consequences.

Transportation

The EAP should include approaches to transport an athlete off the field safely. Medical evacuation to a local emergency care facility may be warranted. A well-designed EAP is devised by the athletic program and local EMS agency. Transportation must encompass the activation of the EMS system, the demarcation of an open route with entry and exit points serviceable to vehicles, the handling and care for the athlete, and the coordination of a standby ambulance for transfer to the nearby medical facility.[20] A member of the sideline medical team must be assigned to accompany the player to the receiving facility.

Venue Location

Every athletic venue needs a site-specific EAP, including a layout of the entire facility with entry and exit points, the location of equipment and communication devices, the position of crucial personnel, accessibility to EMS, and familiarization with the surrounding area and local emergency care facility.[21]

One primary responsibility for the home and away medical teams are coordinating orientation to the site before the game. This provides an overview of the available medical personnel, familiarization with the needs of each medical team, and the most effective course of action in the event of an emergency.[22]

Emergency Care Facilities

The EAP should collaborate between the sports medicine team and the local emergency care facility.[14] These facilities should be notified in advance when an athletic event is occurring. This notice can help with preparation and readiness within the facility to provide a quick, controlled response. This also establishes a direct line of communication between the sideline medical team and facility faculty in the event of injury.

When designing the EAP, the appropriate facility should be designated along with the best routes for transportation. Proximity to the athletic venue should be considered. The facility must be complete with the necessary staff, equipment, and directives to deliver advanced care, including equipment removal.[20] The sideline medical team and the medical facility should review the emergency plan, including clinicians, administrators, and medical staff.

Documentation

During an on-field emergency, the EAP includes documentation that needs to be completed as part of the medical evaluation process. The emergency plan should address the personnel responsible for completing documentation and medical record keeping. These documents and forms need to be readily accessible.

Documentation allows for accountability. This confirms that routine checks of equipment and communication devices are being performed with proper maintenance. Documentation also provides personnel training, qualifications, and certifications that are applicable.

A multiorganizational review of the EAP should be performed annually, including medical personnel, the local care facility, emergency responders, and venue administrators. However, assessments following a rehearsal, or an on-field emergency, should occur more frequently to evaluate for corrections. Any modifications to the EAP should also be a cooperative effort between all contributors.[22]

Emergency Action Plan Pregame Timeout

Time-out is a common term both in athletics and medicine. Time-out in the medical setting is a standardized pause immediately before surgery when all operating room participants stop to verify the procedure, patient identity, correct site, and side. In athletics, coaches and athletes call a time-out to gather the team to discuss strategy or to call a play. The pregame "time-out" is to review the preathletic event checklist and the site-specific EAP.[3] The game day EAP "time-out" is vital in establishing communication and a plan of action in an emergency.

Before the start of each athletic event, an on-field meeting to assemble the athletic health-care professionals should be held. This should include the home and away team physicians, athletic trainers, the on-site EMS, and other medical team members. All athletic health-care team members are introduced, and the chain of command is established. This meeting provides an ideal time to determine the means of communication and how it will occur during an emergency. The time-out offers an ideal time to review the established EAP and determine the role and location of each person present for the event. It identifies the emergency equipment present, its location, and confirmation that it is in working order. This is also the time to determine if an ambulance is on-site as a dedicated unit or on standby. If an ambulance is not on-site, the mechanism for calling one must be addressed. In an emergency requiring transport to a higher level of care, the designated hospital(s) should be selected based on the injury type, necessary treatment, and capabilities of providing appropriate care. Finally, discussions should incorporate the identification and approach for potential same-day issues affecting the EAP, including construction, weather, and crowd flow. The goal of the time-out is to produce a decisive and well-coordinated emergency response to ensure that an injured athlete receives the best care during an emergency.

Review and Improvement

Following each competitive event, the medical team assesses their performance. It is essential for constructive evaluation regarding how the team handled specific scenarios during the event. It also allows the team to critically evaluate its effectiveness during emergent situations and determine areas of improvement. Each on-field event is unique and provides an opportunity for learning and better preparedness the next time the medical health care team is called into action. Attention to small details can make the team more prepared and efficient in the future.

Following the end of the season, a review of the medical health-care performance throughout the season provides an opportunity to optimize the EAP for the future.

SUMMARY

Paramount to the management of on-field emergencies is the foundation of preparation and anticipation. Team physicians should coordinate the establishment and practice of an EAP. Preparation and readiness for on-field emergencies are accomplished through attention to detail and self-assessments. This starts with leadership and communication. A comprehensive EAP that evolves with reviews, a well-educated and devoted medical team, and sufficient rehearsal ensures sideline emergency response competency. Once preparation and readiness are achieved, the team can enjoy the splendor of competition while making a significant difference during an on-field emergency.

CLINICS CARE POINTS

- There is an inherent risk of injury in athletic participation at any level.
- Team medical coverage has evolved and has become a pivotal component of athletics at all levels of competition.
- The goal of a sideline sports medicine team is to prevent injury and manage on-field emergencies.

- An EAP is designed for responding to and treating catastrophic injuries.
- There is a legal basis for an EAP, and the absence has been the basis for negligence claims and lawsuits.
- Prevention starts with preseason physical evaluations to screen for life-threatening conditions and predisposing factors that may contribute to injury or illness.
- Every institution must formulate an EAP developed and reviewed annually by the medical team, administrators, and first responders.
- Preseason training enables the team to practice on-field emergency simulations and develop group cohesion in a low-stress environment.
- Implementation: Achieved through an easy-to-follow written plan, a thoroughly educated team, and rehearsal.
- Personnel: A copy of the EAP should be distributed to all medical personnel, including the team physician, consulting physicians/residents, athletic trainers/students, coaches, and any other member of the sports medicine team.
- Equipment: All equipment should be available at the venue and in operating condition, confirmed by routine checks, and only operated by trained medical personnel.
- Communication: The sideline medical team needs access to a telephone or other communication devices. Communication checks should be completed before each practice and game.
- Transportation: Methods activate the EMS system, handling and care for the athlete, and coordination of a standby ambulance for transfer to the nearby medical facility.
- Venue Location: A site-specific EAP includes a layout of the entire facility with entry and exit points, the location of equipment and communication devices, the position of crucial personnel, accessibility to EMS, and familiarization with the surrounding area and local emergency care facility.
- Emergency Care Facility: The proximity to the athletic venue, capabilities, and directives to deliver advanced care need to be considered.
- Documentation: A part of the medical evaluation process addresses personnel responsible for completing documentation, keeping medical records, and confirming routine checks for equipment and communication devices.
- A pregame time-out aims to produce a decisive and well-coordinated emergency response to provide the best care to an injured athlete during an emergency.
- Following the end of the season, a review of the medical health-care performance throughout the season provides an opportunity to optimize the EAP for the future.

DISCLOSURE

The authors have nothing to disclose.

REFERENCES

1. Niehoff DKL. NFHS handbook. Indianapolis, Indiana: National Federation of State High School Associations; 2019.
2. Kucera K. and Cantu R., Catastrophic sports injury research. Fall 1982 - spring 2018, 2019, National Center for Catastrophic Sports Injury Research At the University of North Carolina at Chapel Hill. Available at: nccsir.unc.edu. October 3, 2019.
3. National athletic trainers' association official statement on athletic health care provider "time outs" before athletic events.

4. Parsons JT, Anderson SA, Casa DJ, et al. Preventing catastrophic injury and death in collegiate athletes: interassociation recommendations endorsed by 13 medical and sports medicine organisations. Br J Sports Med 2020;54(4):208–15.
5. Parsons J. 2014-15 NCAA sports medicine handbook. 25th edition. Indianapolis, Indiana: NCAA Sport Science Institute; 2014.
6. Shultz S, Zinder S, Valovich T. Sports medicine handbook. Indianapolis: National Federation of State High School Associations; 2001.
7. Hedberg R, Messamore W, Poppe T, et al. Emergency action planning in school-based athletics: a systematic review. Kans J Med 2021;14:282–6.
8. Olympia RP, Brady J. Emergency preparedness in high school-based athletics: a review of the literature and recommendations for sport health professionals. Phys Sportsmed 2013;41(2):15–25.
9. Herbert DL. Legal aspects of sports medicine. Canton, OH: Professional Reports Corp; 1990. p. 160–7.
10. MacDonald J, Schaefer M, Stumph J. The preparticipation physical evaluation. Am Fam Physician 2021;103(9):539–46.
11. Miller MD, Thompson SR. Team medical coverage. DeLee, drez, & miller's orthopaedic sports medicine. Philadelphia, PA: Elsevier; 2020. p. 173–84.
12. DeMartini JK, Casa DJ. Who is responsible for preventable deaths during athletic conditioning sessions? J Strength Cond Res 2011;25(7):1781.
13. McDermott ER, Tennent DJ, Patzkowski JC. On-field emergencies and emergency action plans. Sports Med Arthrosc Rev 2021;29(4):e51–6.
14. Casa DJ, Guskiewicz KM, Anderson SA, et al. National athletic trainers' association position statement: preventing sudden death in sports. J Athl Train 2012; 47(1):96–118.
15. Holtzhausen L, Dijkstra HP, Patricios J. Shared decision-making in sports concussion: rise to the 'OCAsion' to take the heat out of on-field decision-making. Br J Sports Med 2019;53(10):590–2.
16. Hainline B, Drezner J, Baggish A, et al. Interassociation consensus statement on cardiovascular care of college student-athletes. Br J Sports Med 2017;51(2): 74–85.
17. Panchal AR, Berg KM, Hirsch KG, et al. 2019 American Heart Association focused update on advanced cardiovascular life support: use of advanced airways, vasopressors, and extracorporeal cardiopulmonary resuscitation during cardiac arrest: an update to the american heart association guidelines for cardiopulmonary resuscitation and emergency cardiovascular care. Circulation 2019; 140(24):e881–94.
18. Emery MS, Kovacs RJ. Sudden cardiac death in athletes. JACC Heart Fail 2018; 6(1):30–40.
19. Herring SA, Kibler W, Putukian M. Sideline preparedness for the team physician: a consensus statement-2012 update. Med Sci Sports Exerc 2012;44(12):2442–5.
20. Courson R, Ellis J, Herring SA, et al. Best practices and current care concepts in prehospital care of the spine-injured athlete in american tackle football march 2-3, 2019; Atlanta, GA. J Athl Train 2020;55(6):545–62.
21. Pelto HF, Drezner JA. Design and implementation of an emergency action plan for sudden cardiac arrest in sport. J Cardiovasc Transl Res 2020;13(3):331–8.
22. Andersen J, Courson RW, Kleiner DM, et al. National athletic trainers' association position statement: emergency planning in athletics. J Athl Train 2002;37(1): 99–104.

The Collapsed Athlete
General Principles

Ryan A. Keenan, MD[a],*, Sourav K. Poddar, MD[b,c],
Alex Ebinger, MD[d], Eric McCarty, MD[e]

KEYWORDS

- Athlete • Sports medicine • Collpased athlete

INTRODUCTION

Sideline management and the ability to assess an athlete's clinical status and presenting symptoms is one of the primary responsibilities of the sports medicine physician. Appropriate medical team coverage requires key skills, planning, and situation-specific training to allow the medical team to provide timely, appropriate, and even potentially life-saving interventions for an athlete's specific condition.

The evaluation of an athlete who is down on the field, course, or other sporting setting by medical staff is unfortunately commonplace during sporting events, although it is usually hidden from the layperson's view by a casual commercial break during televised events. The immediate recognition of a potential emergency and timely response are crucial for a positive outcome. Most of these incidents will be brief and self-resolved, or easily resolved with limited interventions, ending with the athlete being able to ambulate off the field under their own power for further sideline evaluation. However, it is in those situations where the athlete is physically or medically unable to remove themselves under their own power, that emergent evaluation and management by a trained medical staff is essential.

As discussed in earlier articles, the knowledge and presence of an emergency action plan (EAP), as well as the proper rehearsal of said EAP by the medical staff is crucial to the plan's successful implementation and medical management during these rare but critical situations. It is recognized that each sporting discipline will have its own inherent challenges, whether environmental (ie, indoor/outdoor, ice/water/snow sports, ambient temperature, race course logistics), equipment related (ie, helmet, face masks/protective gear, para-athletics, motorsport vehicles), or otherwise. However, the initial evaluation and treatment algorithm necessary for a rapid

No financial disclosures.
[a] University of Colorado School of Medicine, University of Colorado; [b] Department of Family Medicine, University of Colorado School of Medicine, Aurora, CO, USA; [c] Department of Orthopedics, University of Colorado School of Medicine, Aurora, CO, USA; [d] Department of Emergency Medicine, University of Colorado School of Medicine; [e] Department of Orthopedics, University of Colorado School of Medicine, University of Colorado
* Corresponding author.
E-mail address: Ryan.Keenan@cuanschutz.edu

assessment, accurate diagnosis, and appropriate treatment of an athlete's presentation remains implementable across multiple disciplines of sport.

Definitions and Terminology

The "collapsed athlete" is a term commonly referred to throughout sports medicine literature given the multiple urgent and emergent conditions of which the term encompasses. The collapsed athlete has best been defined as an athlete with "failure of a physiologic system (eg, cardiovascular, pulmonary, nervous, or musculoskeletal)" and because of such a failure, the athlete is "unable to continue participating and unable to remove themselves under their own power from the race course or field…".[1,2] Thus, the collapsed athlete encompasses a wide range of clinical presentations, underlying physiology and necessary emergent interventions, subtypes of which will be discussed throughout subsequent articles.

Surveillance data collection and categorization of an athlete's injuries by location, severity, sport, and outcome has been an ongoing and increasingly important effort within the sports medicine research community in order to not only quantify but also use this data in the identification and prevention of future critical injuries and fatalities within the sporting community. The National Center for Catastrophic Sport Injury Research (NCCSIR) collects and analyzes a national database of reported events and athlete-specific injuries in their annual report. As of the 38th annual report, published in September 2022, the cumulative data span the athletic seasons from Fall 1982 to Spring 2021. Within their report, athletic injuries are classified as "fatality," "nonfatal," and "serious," due to the severity and sequelae of the injury ranging from athlete mortality, injury with permanent long-term disability, and severe injury without long-term disability, respectively. Most pertinent to the overall management of the collapsed athlete is the differentiation of the traumatic injury, which they term "direct," that are consequence of the sport-specific skill/actions, and the exertional/medical cohort of "indirect" injuries.[3] Most importantly, the application of this classification system of "direct" and "indirect" injury patterns allows for the initial differentiation within the management algorithm for the collapsed athlete.

DEMOGRAPHICS

There are multiple identifiable risk factors that may play a role in the predilection of an athlete to collapse and require acute medical attention, including but not limited to.

- The overall fitness level of the athlete
- Hydration/nutrition status, concurrent illness
- Medication use (such as insulin, opioids, and stimulants such as amphetamines or cocaine)
- Individual medical history (sickle cell trait or disease, history of exertional syncope, or congenital contributors)
- Family history of predisposing factors and conditions.
- Environmental factors (wet-bulb globe readings, allergen exposures, lightning, rapid weather changes)
- And ultimately the conditions within a competition that may lead to overexertion (pushing past discomfort and safety for competitive or goal-oriented reasons, such as in elite competition or fitness testing scenarios).

During the past 3 decades, the total athlete population and participation numbers have notably increased at all competition levels, sports, and within athletic populations. The overall participation is measured in athlete-seasons due to the potential for a single athlete to compete in multiple sports during a given year, or even season. Both the National Federation of State High School Associations (NFHS) and the National Collegiate Athletics Association (NCAA) have noted an increased participation in their yearly surveys over time (acknowledging the limited sport participation in the Spring/Fall 2020 seasons due to pandemic cancellations). During the 2020 and 2021 seasons, the NFHS estimated total high school participation at 7,618,054 (57.4% men), whereas the NCAA noted 491,255 athlete seasons (56.1% men) in championship sports.[4,5] This number underestimates the participation given not all schools are members of the NFHS and NCAA, leading to a statistically underreported total participation within the United States. Given this ongoing growth of sport and gross increase in athlete-seasons on a year-to-year basis, it would be logical to expect an increased total incidence of athlete-related injury and potentially fatal events, despite the relatively low frequency of events.

Sports-related deaths and nonfatal catastrophic injuries are becoming increasingly rare. This is due in part to innovations in equipment safety technology, changes to sport-specific protocols and rules within regulatory bodies, paired with an increased prevalence of dedicated medical coverage during high-risk events. However, they do still occur. A well-known example of one such rule change is the outlawing of "spear tackling," the act of leading with the crown of the head in American football. This has led to a reported decrease in axial spine injury/debility at all levels over the following years and the subsequent "Heads-up Football" campaign. The program, led by USA Football, teaches coaches the proper approach to training youth athletes in tackling technique and, even further, the management of potential emergencies in youth football.

Despite these direct efforts to increase safety within sport at all levels, the most recent 2022 NCCSIR Annual Report, noted 2958 sport-related catastrophic events over the 39 years of data collection (60 in 2020–2021 alone), the majority of which have been nonfatal (64%) traumatic "direct" mechanisms (63%) within high school athletes (79%). During their analysis they noted similar data trends within high school and collegiate athletes, traumatic/indirect ratio, and fatal versus nonfatal, with incidence being highest in football versus other sports at both levels of play (noting greatest overall participation rate). In addition to American football, when participation rates (per 100,000 athlete seasons) were considered, sports such as cheerleading, gymnastics, ice hockey, and skiing had the highest rates of catastrophic injuries.[3]

Initial Approach to the Collapsed Athlete

The initial management of the collapsed athlete is founded in the fundamental principles of basic life support (BLS). The initiation of the advanced cardiac life support (ACLS) and/or advanced trauma life support (ATLS) treatment algorithms may be warranted depending on the level of training of the medical staff and the unique presentation of the patient. These systems are the basis for the initial evaluation and resuscitation of critical conditions, such as cardiac arrest and traumatic arrest. However, advanced interventions should never delay timely BLS interventions. Initiation of advanced interventions should be evaluated on a case-by-case basis due to sideline limitations, which include but are not limited to training level of the medical team, access to resources/medications, and environmental determinants.

Scene Safety

Before patient evaluation and treatment initiation, the use of personal protective equipment (PPE), and the evaluation of scene safety is crucial to the safety of the medical team and the athlete in question. Each coverage environment will pose unique safety hazards that need to be identified (a notable component of a well thought out EAP) and controlled before safely activating and mobilizing the medical team. For example, motorsports may require a pause in racing, evacuation of the athlete from dangers, or clearance of hazardous material before evaluation. Large endurance events may require crowd control or course diversion of athletes to allow for medical response, and downhill snow events may require waiting for other athletes to clear the course. Scene safety is of utmost importance given the speed with which a single athlete evaluation could turn into a mass casualty event (simply defined as when patients outnumber the resources available) if a member of the medical team were to become injured during a medical response. Not only would this divide resources to address both patients but also is compounded by the loss of key medical personnel within the proposed and rehearsed action plan. In primarily environmental sources of injury, such as in lightning strikes, the initiation of treatment at the scene (on the X) versus moving the patient to safety before treatment (load and go) should be addressed based on scene safety and the EAP/local emergency medical services (EMS) protocol. Given the diversity of sporting events and locations, each unique environment will necessitate its own protocols and risk analysis in order to make the scene the safest possible for both the athlete and the responding medical team.

Immediate EMS Activation: Responsive Versus Unresponsive Versus Acute Decompensating

After verification of scene safety, the primary survey differentiates the responsive patient from the unresponsive/critically ill patient. As is taught in ACLS and ATLS, the primary survey consisting of airway, breathing, and circulation (ABC) is key to the early identification and management of life-threatening conditions. This assessment can be expanded to include principles of the MARCH protocol, in order to control massive hemorrhage before airway and breathing evaluation, "C→AB."

MARCH protocol

M, massive hemorrhage
A, airway
R, respiration
C, circulation
H, hypothermia/head injury

MARCH is a key protocol within the tactical field care phase of Tactical Combat Casualty Care (TCCC or TC3) and has been linked to a decrease in the overall fatality of battlefield injuries since its initial institution during the early 2000s.[6] In battlefield data, acute hemorrhage was identified as the primary cause of death in 91% of cases studied, in comparison with 7.9% noted to be airway related.[7] This identifiable trend in battlefield deaths, lead to the development, and subsequent success of the MARCH protocol due to the prioritization of controlling acute hemorrhage before the traditional emphasis on a secure airway. Although collapsed athletes are not typically prone to the same penetrating battlefield injuries seen in the warfighter population, they may present with acute life-threatening bleeding, such as in acute hockey skate lacerations. Due to the overlap of battlefield and civilian presentations, key elements of TCCC have been increasingly adapted within civilian EMS protocols and training during the past decade. These critical interventions are increasingly prevalent in first-responder trainings, and even courses directed at the general population with programs such as "Stop the Bleed," which aims to teach the general public principles of the immediate response to life-threatening bleeding through wound packing and proper tourniquet use. Techniques for the management of acute hemorrhage/vascular injuries will be discussed in a future article.

Notably, BLS resuscitation (early cardiopulmonary resuscitation [CPR] initiation, automated external defibrillator (AED) retrieval, and attachment/activation with early activation of the EAP or EMS system via 911) should occur in any athlete who is initially found to be.

1. *Unresponsive* (no eye opening to voice, no movement, or localizing pain response)
2. *Pulseless* (or an irregular nonperfusing pulse)
   and/or
3. *Apneic* (not breathing) or agonal respirations (non-life-sustaining breaths)

It is important to note that AED availability and use within 3 to 5 minutes of initial arrest has been identified as one of the most effective interventions for cardiac arrest.[8] Its timely implementation has increased the overall functional survival rate for cardiac arrest patients nearly 20% during the course of a decade (2000–2010).[9] If a trained ACLS/ATLS provider is present, early interventions for reversible causes can be attempted following initiation and continuation of the BLS protocol; however, these interventions should not delay emergency activation of EMS/AED and/or transport to an emergency department for definitive treatment, if indicated.

The in-depth approach to unresponsive and acutely altered mental status presentations from various causes will be covered in subsequent articles; however, the differential diagnosis should include elements such as sudden cardiac arrest; exertional heat/cold illness; respiratory arrest; severe electrolyte derangements such as hyponatremia; insulin shock/hypoglycemia; exertional collapse associated with sickle cell trait (ECAST); in addition to major trauma (commotion cordis, hemorrhage, blunt traumatic injury…). The initial evaluation can be further condensed into the "3 H's" … "Head (trauma), Heat, and Heart," 3 of the most common emergent sideline presentations requiring directed management.

RESPONSIVE PATIENT, FOCUSED HISTORY AND PHYSICAL

Once the mental and cardiac statuses of the patient have been evaluated and determined to be noncritical, further management should be guided by a focused history and physical examination. This focused evaluation should include elements of a "SAMPLE" history as described below while obtaining a directed physical examination and vital signs.

SAMPLE History

(S) Signs (Observed respiratory rate (RR), HR palpation, BP when able, Temp (core required if altered mental status)
S Symptoms—Symptoms preceding the event and current symptoms: chest pain, airway/SOB, neurovascular changes, nausea, vomiting, and musculoskeletal pain
A Allergies (if applicable—anaphylaxis—remove offending agent/decon)
M Medications—Daily, stimulants/supplements, insulin pump
P Past medical History (PMHx)—(known medical conditions: asthma, diabetes, cardiac factors, congenital heart/family hx of heart disease)
L Last meal, hydration, or nutrition regimen—(too little or too many electrolytes)
E Events leading up to presentation: potential direct (traumatic) versus indirect (medical cause)

Dependent on setting and the quantity of medical services/resources available, adjunct testing such as point of care glucose, electrolyte measurements (sodium, potassium), and indwelling core thermometers may be indicated to guide diagnosis and subsequent interventions.

Initiate Treatment of Identified Etiology

If a primary cause of collapse is identified by the focused HPI and physical examination, initiation of the appropriate interventions is indicated based on the qualifications of the medical team, available resources, and potential for decompensation before transport to definitive management. Although there is a wide differential diagnosis for collapsed athletes, the approach can be simplified by mechanism, organ system, and pathologic condition.

Each of the following life-threatening conditions will be addressed in future articles; however, the basic tenets of early activation of the EAP/EMS, and stabilization of life-threats while awaiting transport, remain crucial to positive outcomes.

Trauma

- The "direct" traumatic injury encompasses the care of conditions directly due to the cause of the sport and typically originates from a collision/contact with another player or environmental factors. The acute management of traumatic injuries requires early identification and interventions, whether head trauma (ie, acute facial injuries or ICH/seizure… to be discussed in Jessica Tsao and Calvin Eric Hwang's article, "Emergency Facial Injuries in Athletics"; and Ashwin L. Rao and colleagues' article, "Head Injuries and Emergencies in Sports," in this issue), spinal trauma (see Ron Courson and colleagues' article, "Acute and Emergent Spinal Injury Assessment and Treatment," in this issue), intrathoracic trauma (ie, pneumo/hemothorax, vascular injury…see Alexander J. Tomesch and colleagues' article, "Chest and Thorax Injuries in Athletes," in this issue), intra-abdominal trauma (ie, solid organ and hollow viscous injury… see Ross E. Mathiasen and Christopher P. Hogrefe's article, "Emergency Abdominopelvic Injuries," in this issue), or extremity trauma (ie, active hemorrhage, dislocation, fracture, compartment syndromes… see James T. Stannard and James P. Stannard's article, "Fractures and Dislocations on the Playing Field: Which Are Emergent and What to Do?"; and Omar Farah and colleagues' article, "Acute Compartment Syndrome in the Athlete," in this issue). Acute traumatic injuries should be treated with heightened awareness for concomitant neck injuries and implement spinal precautions such as c-spine stabilization, log rolls, and team lifts early in evaluation until the athlete can be fully evaluated and cleared.

Cardiac

- The differential for cardiac collapse is broad, encompassing topics from sudden cardiac arrest, arrhythmia, acute cardiac syndrome (heart attack), congenital causes such as arrhythmogenic right ventricular dysplasia (ARVD)/Brugada/ and hypertrophic cardiomyopathy to benign conditions such as exercise associated postural hypotension (EAPH). For the presumed cardiac arrest, BLS and AED ± ACLS remain the critical initial steps in the management linked to positive outcomes.
- EAPH remains solely as a diagnosis of exclusion within the subgroup of cardiac associated collapse. EAPH can be summarized as collapse secondary to the transient loss of blood return/preload to the heart. Cardiac preload is aided by the "second heart" phenomenon, the rhythmic contraction of lower body muscles during exercise, which is lost immediately following secession of exercise

when the contracting leg muscles are no longer helping to return blood to the heart. This decrease in blood return to the right heart is paired with a transient inability for baroreceptors to compensate, leading to near syncope/athlete collapse. This loss of preload is commonly treated with the leg raised or "recovery position," and recovery occurs quickly once the body is able to equilibrate. Athletes with EAPH (typically endurance after marathon) are usually able to be cleared with no need for intravenous (IV) fluids or transfer to a higher level of care.

Respiratory

- Primary respiratory complications include airway obstructions, such as a mouthpiece, and asthma exacerbations both atopic and potentially exercise induced/environmental. Asthmatic presentations are typically characterized by poor airflow, an expiratory wheeze, with or without a preceding diagnosis of asthma. Sideline management should be guided by appearance and symptoms severity. Acute obstruction relief can be with attempted through the removal of foreign body with finger sweep, Heimlich maneuver, or device assisted. Additionally, albuterol inhalers and supplemental oxygen (if available) can be used to initially manage asthma exacerbations before disposition decisions.

Environmental

- Environmental factors can have a significant impact on athlete performance, whether through hypothermia/hyperthermia (heat illness to heat stroke), altitude (eg, acute mountain sickness, high altitude pulmonary or cerebral [HACE] edema), lightning strikes, or injuries related to the competition setting (eg, ice friction burns in luge/skeleton or drowning in triathletes). A key point of management in EHS—exertional heat stroke (heat plus altered mental status)—patients is the need to "cool first, transport second," given the fact that prolonged time at supraphysiologic temperatures has been linked to cognitive and long-term negative outcomes The most recent consensus statement on EHS supports this protocol given the fact that "when cooling is delayed, there is a significant increase in organ damage, morbidity, and mortality after 30 minutes, faster than the average EMS transport and emergency department evaluation window."[10]

Metabolic/endocrine

- Prolonged endurance activity predisposes athletes to metabolic derangements most commonly presenting as hyponatremia/hypernatremia, dependent on inherent fluid/salt losses, hydration status, and exogenous salt replacement throughout the course of the event. The availability of a point of care device for testing would allow for increased diagnostic certainty and could guide treatment based on severity.

Additionally, exercise-induced hypoglycemia is predominantly seen in patients with underlying diabetes/endocrinopathies, or coinciding illness. Insulin shock can manifest as a critical presentation of hypoglycemia, although typically seen in patient with known type 1 diabetes and on long-acting insulins or indwelling pumps. Initial management centers in the removal of the offending agent, typically a malfunctioning pump, and glucose replacement in the form of food by mouth or IV dextrose in severe presentations.

Hematologic

- There are limited emergent hematologic presentations for the collapsed athlete. One of the most notable, ECAST—exercise collapse associated with sickle cell trait (SCT), is an increasingly demonstrated cause of acute athlete collapse in patients with SCT. The pathologic condition of ECAST stems from exercise causing a local inflammatory response in muscle tissue, relative local hypoxia, and increased temperatures coupled with relative dehydration. These physiologic changes at the cellular level lead to a downstream metabolic acidosis within the tissue and microvascular environments. Given the shift in the oxygen dissociation curve with pH shift, coupled with an increasingly anaerobic environment, there is a potential for increased sickling and microvascular occlusion, ultimately leading to skeletal muscle failure, potassium shifts and the potential for sudden cardiac arrest if not addressed. This may additionally present as exertional compartment syndrome before critical presentations. This diagnosis should be on the differential in any patient who may possess the sickle cell trait given the potential for acute decompensation, and will likely need acute management at a higher level of care.

Allergic

- Athletes may self-present with allergies in various settings, whether as a sequalae of an insect bite or sting, or contact with/ingestion of a known or unknown allergen. It is important to differentiate the localized allergic response from a true anaphylactic emergency. This distinction can be made through the presents of multisystem involvement, as opposed to isolated skin/localized findings, with or without known allergen exposure. Anaphylaxis remains in the list of critical diagnoses of the collapsed athlete, whether alert or unresponsive; however, patients will typically present in respiratory distress with signs of additional multisystem involvement (inspiratory stridor, cardiac collapse, diffuse urticarial rash, nausea/vomiting, or diarrhea). Immediate intervention with IM epinephrine, commonly referred to as an epi-pen, is indicated for the acute avoidance of cardiac collapse or arrest and progression of illness severity. In the event that an epi-pen is given, it is likely that the patient will require transport to be evaluated due to the potential recurrence of symptoms or further decompensation in respiratory or cardiac status.

Pharmacologic

- With the increasing prevalence of opioid use, both prescribed and nonprescribed, there is an increasing incidence of accidental overdose and fatalities within both the general population and the sports community. Although there have been multiple federal and state programs aimed at harm reduction and social mitigation of drug use, it remains as one of the leading, and rapidly growing, causes of avoidable death in the United States.[11] Given the prevalence within the general population, it is not unprecedented to add opioid overdose to the differential of the collapsed athlete with associated respiratory depression, apnea or even in events of atypical cardiac arrests. Nasal naloxone, a competitive opioid antagonist, can be an immediate and directly lifesaving intervention when indicated and is an important addition to a sideline medical kit in case of athlete or bystander emergencies.

SUMMARY

The collapsed athlete encompasses multiple critical and noncritical pathologic conditions, management of which highly depends on the elements of presentation of an athlete, the environment in which the athlete presents, and the key history elements leading to the collapse. In all collapsed athletes, early identification of an unresponsive/pulseless athlete with prompt BLS/CPR, AED use, and EMS activation is key, with the addition of early hemorrhage control in acute traumatic injuries. Once the primary survey is cleared, the initiation of a focused history and physical examination is critical to rule out life-threatening causes of collapse and to further guide initial management and disposition.

CLINICS CARE POINTS

- Scene safety, PPE, and early activation of EMS/the EAP are critical to efficient and appropriate care for the collapsed athlete.
- Immediate triage should involve mental status (unresponsive vs responsive) and ABC's.
- In the event of an unresponsive/pulseless patient immediate BLS/ACLS/ATLS should be initiated.
- BLS (CPR/AED) should never be delayed for advanced interventions.
- AED activation and use within 3 to 5 minutes has been linked to increased survival rates.
- In the responsive patient a targeted history and physical examination is likely to identify underlying reason for collapse and emergent interventions/management.
- Low threshold for C-spine/immobilization if there is a concern for traumatic injury.
- Acute cooling should be completed before transport in the event of acute hyperthermia/heat stroke.
- EAPH is a diagnosis of exclusion, given multiple life-threatening diagnoses that must first be ruled out/evaluated.

REFERENCES

1. O'Connor FG, Brennan FH. Evaluation of the collapsed adult athlete. UpToDate. Updated: July 06, 2022. Available at: https://www.uptodate.com/contents/evaluation-of-the-collapsed-adult-athlete. Accessed November 6, 2022.
2. Asplund CA, O'Connor FG, Noakes TD. Exercise-associated collapse: an evidence-based review and primer for clinicians. Br J Sports Med 2011;45(14):1157–62.
3. Kucera KL, Cantu RC, National Center for Catastrophic Sport Injury Research-38th Annual Report. Available at: https://nccsir.unc.edu/wp-content/uploads/sites/5614/2022/10/2021-Catastrophic-Report-AS-39th-AY2020-2021-FINALw.pdf. Accessed November 5, 2022.
4. National Federation of State High School Associations, (NFHS), 2021-22 High School Athletics Participation Survey, Online PDF Available at: https://www.nfhs.org/sports-resource-content/high-school-participation-survey-archive/. Accessed November 1, 2022.
5. NCAA, NCAa sports sponsorship and participation rates report: 2020-21 update, Online PDF Available at: https://ncaaorg.s3.amazonaws.com/research/sportpart/2021RES_SportsSponsorshipParticipationRatesReport.pdf. Accessed November 1, 2022.
6. Butler FK, Holcomb JB, Giebner SD, et al. Tactical combat casualty care 2007: evolving concepts and battlefield experience. Mil Med 2007;172(11 Suppl):1–19.

7. Eastridge BJ, Mabry RL, Seguin P, et al. Death on the battlefield (2001-2011): implications for the future of combat casualty care. J Trauma Acute Care Surg 2012; 73(6 Suppl 5):S431–7.

8. Courson R. Preventing sudden death on the athletic field: the emergency action plan. Curr Sports Med Rep 2007;6:93–100.

9. Maron BJ. Estes, commotio cordis. N Engl J Med 2010;362:917–27.

10. Belval LN, Casa DJ, Adams WM, et al. Consensus statement- prehospital care of exertional heat stroke. Prehosp Emerg Care 2018;22(3):392–7.

11. Mattson CL, Tanz LJ, Quinn K, et al. Trends and geographic patterns in drug and synthetic opioid overdose deaths — United States, 2013–2019. MMWR Morb Mortal Wkly Rep 2021;70:202–7.

Cardiac Emergency in the Athlete

William Denq, MD, CAQ-SM[a],*, Ben Oshlag, MD, CAQ-SM[b]

KEYWORDS

- Cardiac emergency • Cardiac arrest • Collapsed athlete • Arrhythmia • CPR
- Cardiomyopathy

KEY POINTS

- Timely quality chest compressions and time to defibrillation are the greatest factors affecting survival in cardiac arrest.
- Initial management of cardiac emergencies includes activation of emergency medical services (EMS), early cardiopulmonary resuscitation (CPR), rapid defibrillation, and transfer to an appropriate medical center.
- Sudden cardiac arrest should be suspected in any collapsed and unresponsive athlete, and an automated external defibrillator (AED) should be used as early as possible, with CPR taking place until it can be applied.
- Underlying cardiac abnormalities that can predispose some athletes to sudden cardiac arrest include cardiomyopathies, coronary artery anomalies, and channelopathies, as well as genetic disorders such as sickle cell trait, and Marfan syndrome.
- Formal planning for an efficient response and effective care can help avoid catastrophic outcomes.

INTRODUCTION, BACKGROUND, AND PREVALENCE

Cardiac-related deaths are the leading nontraumatic cause of death in the young athlete and second leading cause overall behind accidents. Earlier estimates on the incidence of sudden cardiac death (SCD) varied widely, ranging from 1:3000 athlete-years (AY) to 1:917,000 AY but more recent studies have shown a rate of approximately 1:50,000 AY in collegiate athletes and 1:50,000 to 1:80,000 AY in high school athletes. The highest risk groups include men, black athletes, and basketball players, with Division I male black basketball players being found to have approximately 1:4000 AY risk.[1] Soccer and football players were also found to be among the highest risk athletes. These athletes are typically healthy at baseline but may have undiagnosed conditions that put them at an elevated risk for

[a] University of Arizona, 1501 North Campbell Avenue, Tucson, P.O. Box 245057, AZ 85724, USA;
[b] White Plains Hospital, 41 East Post Road, White Plains, NY 10601, USA
* Corresponding author. 1501 N. Campbell Avenue, Tucson, P.O. Box 245057, AZ 85724.
E-mail address: denq@arizona.edu

Clin Sports Med 42 (2023) 355–371
https://doi.org/10.1016/j.csm.2023.02.003
0278-5919/23/© 2023 Elsevier Inc. All rights reserved.
sportsmed.theclinics.com

dangerous cardiac events, including cardiomyopathies, coronary artery anomalies (CAAs), or channelopathies. Due to the nature of the patient population involved, the social, health, and economic impacts of SCD are significant.[2] This has led to extensive research into preparticipation screening examinations and diagnostic tools to try to uncover these conditions before they lead to catastrophic outcomes. Despite this, cardiac events can and do still occur on a regular basis, and preparation and prompt evaluation and treatment are vital because planning for effective care to respond to cardiac emergencies can help avoid catastrophic outcomes.

Prompt evaluation and treatment of a cardiac arrest patient is crucial to their chances for meaningful long-term survival. The greatest factor affecting survival is the time between arrest and initial defibrillation, with survival rates of up to 74% if defibrillated within 3 minutes, whereas only 49% if defibrillated after 3 minutes,[3] and rates declining by 7% to 10% with every minute that defibrillation is delayed.[4] Timely bystander cardiopulmonary resuscitation (CPR) can also significantly improve outcomes, even in situations with prolonged EMS response time.[5]

In this article, we will discuss cardiac emergencies in athletes, with a primary focus on evaluation and management of on-the-field cardiac events. We will discuss the most common causes of sudden cardiac arrest, and the underlying pathophysiology of these disorders. We will also discuss the long-term management of athletes with these conditions, including postarrest care and return to play considerations.

APPROACH TO THE COLLAPSED ATHLETE

Case Vignette: An 18-year-old football player is seen to collapse while running a play. He is not responsive on arrival.

Overall approach: Regardless of inciting cause, this is a case of witnessed arrest until proven otherwise. The approach is the same: early recognition of an emergency, scene safety, EMS activation, early CPR, early defibrillation if indicated, and rapid transition to advanced life support.[6] It is important to be familiar with any established emergency action plan (EAP) for the venue to avoid any confusion and mismanagement of care.

Scene safety: Ensure that the environment is safe to render aid. Be cognizant of the surroundings, whether it be teammates, the crowd, vehicles, or nature (eg, lightning strikes).

Evaluation: On the initial approach to the collapsed athlete, it is crucial to follow the basic life support (BLS) sequence as recommended by the International Liaison Committee on Resuscitation.[6,7]

Management and stabilization: Initiation of CPR is recommended in the witnessed collapsed athlete regardless of whether cardiac arrest is the cause for collapse.[6] The steps are adapted from the original article as follows for a health-care provider after determining scene safety.

1. Assess for response.
2. If no response, activate EMS.
3. Check for apnea or agonal breathing and check for pulses simultaneously. Prepare to begin compressions.
   a. AED/emergency equipment should be retrieved immediately after the check by a second responder
4. If apneic or agonal breathing, immediately begin CPR. Second responder should apply pads from the AED/defibrillator when available.
5. As soon as AED/defibrillator is available, pause CPR to administer shock.

6. Immediately resume CPR after shock administration and perform 2-person CPR with the second responder.
7. Compressions to ventilation are 30:2.[a]

Compressions: Quality chest compressions are crucial for proper cardiac arrest management in the collapsed athlete. Chest compression depth and rate are the 2 most important factors when determining the quality of chest compressions. Chest compressions of 2 inches (5 cm) to 2.4 inches (6 cm) and a rate of 100 to 120 compressions/min are optimal. A pulse check of the carotid artery should be performed every 2 minutes with minimal interruption to compressions.[9] Chest compressions are known to be affiliated with sternal fractures, rib fractures, hemopneumothorax, and other traumatic injuries.

AED: On AED arrival and pad placement, a shock should be delivered if advised.

It is important to note that these steps are for a health-care provider but different for a trained or untrained layperson. Please refer to BLS guidelines.

SPECIAL CONSIDERATIONS

CPR-induced consciousness: This increasingly reported phenomenon occurs in 0.23% to 0.9% of CPR attempts.[10] During CPR, the athlete may become combative, begin groaning, or even open their eyes. However, with cessation of CPR and, subsequently, cerebral perfusion, the athlete will become unresponsive and lose pulses. There is no clear guidance on the benefit of sedation or analgesia but there are reports of fast-acting medications such as fentanyl, midazolam, or ketamine being used to help reduce the pain and trauma associated with CPR.[10] However, it is of the utmost importance that CPR be continued until the athlete has proper return of spontaneous circulation (ROSC).

Exercise-related collapse in the athlete with sickle cell trait: Of special importance, high flow oxygen in an athlete with exercise-related collapse in the athlete with sickle cell trait (ECAST) has a theoretic benefit in reducing sickling associated with hypoxia.[11] However, as mentioned above, high flow oxygen should already be administered in a cardiac resuscitation.

Lightning strike: In the event of a lightning strike, one or multiple athletes can be struck. Unlike other mass casualty events, lightning strike victims should be reverse triaged. Typically, those who are in cardiac arrest are "black tagged" and resources are directed to those who exhibit signs of life. However, in a lightning strike, a reverse triage system is used.[12] Victims that seem dead should be the first to receive treatment in the form of CPR because these victims will likely regain spontaneous automaticity or have a reversible arrhythmia.[12] If ROSC is achieved, respiratory support may be needed until spontaneous respirations return. Victims of a lightning strike that survive immediately after the event are unlikely to have significant mortality before transfer to a higher level of care. It should be noted that although this article only discusses cardiac system-related issues, there are other involved systems after a lightning strike.[12] In the solo athlete, proceed with approach to the collapsed athlete algorithm.

---

[a] Chest compression only CPR performed by bystanders in out-of-hospital cardiac arrest patients has been shown to be superior to standard CPR where rescue breaths are given.[8] About 13.3% of cardiac arrest victims survive with compression only CPR compared with 7.8% with standard CPR.[8] The reasoning is that ventilation interrupts proper organ perfusion. A nonrebreather mask at 15 L can be used to passively ventilate the patient while compressions can be performed without pause.

PATHOPHYSIOLOGY

There is a multitude of causes for cardiac arrest in the athlete. The following are a select number of important causes pertinent to sideline cardiac collapse. Signs and symptoms preceding collapse are reviewed as well.

HYPERTROPHIC CARDIOMYOPATHY

Hypertrophic cardiomyopathy (HCM) is a genetically induced left ventricular hypertrophy without other secondary causes. Typically asymmetric, it is often most severe in the intraventricular septum and histologically shows myocyte hypertrophy, disarray, and interstitial fibrosis. This can result in left ventricular outflow tract obstruction. Patients typically have nondilated left ventricles and a normal to increased ejection fraction and can also have diastolic dysfunction. Most HCM is asymptomatic but can present with chest pain, arrhythmia, syncope, or sudden cardiac arrest. Symptoms are secondary to myocardial hypoperfusion that results from reduced blood flow through thick-walled coronary arteries, as well as increased oxygen demand from hypertrophied myocardium. This can lead to nonsustained ventricular tachycardia, ventricular fibrillation, and cardiac arrest.[13]

ARRHYTHMOGENIC RIGHT VENTRICULAR CARDIOMYOPATHY

Arrhythmogenic right ventricular cardiomyopathy (ARVC) is a genetically heterogenous disease characterized pathologically by the replacement of normal myocardium with fibrofatty tissue and clinically by ventricular arrhythmias and dysfunction. The change in tissue results in wall thinning and aneurysm formation in the ventricles. Wall thinning can also result in ventricular dysfunction, often starting with the right ventricle due to its thinner wall. This can progress to biventricular dysfunction at end-stage disease. Exercise, especially endurance sports, can accelerate wall thinning. As a result, AC is a leading cause for sudden cardiac death (SCD).[14]

DILATED CARDIOMYOPATHY

Dilated cardiomyopathy is characterized by a dilated left ventricle with systolic dysfunction that is not caused by ischemic or valvular heart disease. Ventricular remodeling occurs, driven by pathologic myocyte hypertrophy, myocyte apoptosis, myofibroblast proliferation, and interstitial fibrosis. The alteration in ventricular architecture leads to an increased chamber volume, and the dilation of the left or both ventricles causes reduced systolic function with an increased preload but reduced stroke volume and contractility. Patients with dilated cardiomyopathy can develop a broad range of atrial and ventricular arrhythmias that can lead to collapse or sudden cardiac arrest.[15]

BRUGADA

Brugada syndrome is an electrical cardiac disorder that predisposes patients to SCD through the development of ventricular tachycardia and ventricular fibrillation in a structurally normal heart. The arrhythmias are secondary to mutations in cardiac ion channels that alter the transmembrane ion currents that constitute the cardiac action potential. Variants in 19 genes have been implicated but it is not known how much each of these contribute to clinical disease, and whether Brugada is caused by changes to depolarization, repolarization, or current-load match is a question still under debate.[16] The mutations lead to diagnostic electrocardiogram

(ECG) changes with right ventricular conduction delay, coved-shaped or saddle-shaped ST segment elevation, and/or T-wave inversion. This alters the excitation wavelength, which ultimately increases the risk of arrhythmia, syncope, and sudden death. Most individuals are asymptomatic, and it is not known what factors predispose to arrhythmia, although the risk of recurrence after an initial episode is approximately 50%. Ventricular fibrillation occurs more often at night during periods of increased vagal tone, although fever and certain drugs can also increase the risk.[17,18]

MYOCARDITIS

Myocarditis is an inflammatory disease of the myocardium that occurs in 3 phases: acute viral, subacute immune, and chronic phase.[19] The acute phase is commonly associated with a viral infection, although there are noninfectious causes such as autoimmune conditions (inflammatory bowel disease, rheumatoid arthritis, and so forth) or pharmacologic induced (antibiotics, amphetamines, anabolic agents, and so forth).[20] Athletes are particularly susceptible to myocarditis when traveling, competing in extreme environments, and pushing past physical limits—all potential reasons for a compromised immune system, which increases the risk for viral infection. The acute viral phase may often go undetected because it is short lived but the following subacute and chronic inflammation stages can result in the destruction of myocytes and improper cardiac remodeling. This remodeling can result in an increased risk of arrhythmia. Endurance athletes can trigger a more significant inflammatory response, which may magnify the potential for arrhythmia. After recovery, a chronic cycle of cytokine inflammation may persist. Overall, these factors make myocarditis one of the leading causes of sudden death in athletes.

Similar to other viruses, direct infiltration of SARS-CoV-2 into the myocardium produces a strong cytokine response resulting in complications such as arrhythmias and SCD.[21]

Myocarditis in the acute phase is often a mild presentation of vague symptoms that are variable from case to case. If a viral illness is the cause, it can present with symptoms such as fevers, rigors, rhinorrhea, cough, nausea, vomiting, headache, palpitations, myalgias, shortness of breath, or lightheadedness. If the athlete reports chest pain or other cardiac symptoms (eg, syncope), have an increased index of suspicion for myocarditis.

CORONARY ARTERY ANOMALIES

SCD associated with CAAs occur mostly during exercise. An anomalous coronary artery with an aortic origin is one of the most common causes of SCD in the athlete.[22,23] However, it is not the only anomaly reported—there are a vast number of other CAAs. To simplify this, the anomalies can be divided into 3 categories: anomalies of origin, course, and termination.

Anomalies of origin: Athletes with an anomalous pulmonary origin of the coronary arteries may suffer from ischemia in affected myocardial territories.[23] The level of ischemia may depend on oxygen demand and collateral circulation. About 17% of athletes with an anomalous pulmonary origin of the left coronary artery have either ventricular arrhythmia or SCD.[23]

Anomalies of course: Myocardial bridging occurs when a coronary artery courses intramurally within the heart. It is often associated with a higher risk of myocardial infarction. High-grade stenosis of the coronary ostium should be considered as a risk for heart failure and potential SCD.[23]

Anomalies of termination: Coronary fistulas typically result in right-sided heart failure or chronic dyspnea but SCD is only theoretic possibility.[23]

Dyspnea and exertional chest pain typically occur first. However, SCD may be the first presentation of CAA. This is estimated to occur in up to 50% of cases.[23]

The diagnostic gold standard for CAA IS coronary computed tomography angiography.[22] ECG, echocardiogram, and stress test are other important diagnostics to consider especially when evaluating from ischemic disease caused by CAAs.[23]

SICKLE COLLAPSE (EXERCISE-RELATED COLLAPSE IN THE ATHLETE WITH SICKLE CELL TRAIT)

The mechanism of ECAST is not completely understood. However, it is known that the risk of exercise-related death in Division 1 athletes is 37 times higher in SCT athletes compared with athletes without SCT.[24] A commonly proposed theory is that vigorous exercise can result in hyperthermia and dehydration triggering vaso-occlusion and endothelial damage from hemoglobin S polymerization. This vaso-occlusive crisis reduces blood flow and increases cellular destruction. A cascade of rhabdomyolysis, hyperkalemia, increasing acidosis, disseminated intravascular coagulation, cardiac and renal failure, and arrhythmia can occur. Poor conditioning, high ambient temperatures, dehydration, or altitude can be risk factors for a sickle collapse in an SCT athlete.[25,26]

ECAST may initially present as a "conscious collapse" where the athlete is listless but still conversant. They often report weakness more than pain. Alternatively, acute collapses have been reported.[11]

STABLE VERSUS UNSTABLE TACHYARRHYTHMIAS

Tachyarrhythmias are abnormal heart rhythms in which the heart is beating faster than usual. Causes can vary widely but can generally be broken down into atrial and ventricular tachycardias. Clinically, it is also important to differentiate between stable and unstable tachyarrhythmias because the treatment differs significantly between the two. Atrial tachycardias include atrioventricular reentrant tachycardia, atrioventricular nodal reentrant tachycardia, atrial fibrillation, atrial flutter, and Wolff-Parkinson-White syndrome. These tachyarrhythmias initiate in the atria and typically involve premature beats triggering a reentrant circuit. This circuit repeatedly generates ventricular beats, which bypass the rate control of the AV node and can generate heart rates as high as 250 to 300 bpm. The location of the circuit, as well as typical ECG findings, differentiates the atrial tachyarrhythmias. Ventricular tachyarrhythmias include ventricular tachycardia and ventricular fibrillation. These rhythms are much more likely to be unstable and are the most common causes of SCD. Ventricular tachycardia is a wide-complex tachycardia that can be sustained or nonsustained, depending on the duration, and monomorphic or polymorphic, based on the QRS morphology. The mechanism involves enhancement of normal or abnormal automaticity, early or late depolarizations, and reentry circuits, whereas causes can include ischemic heart disease, structural abnormalities, channelopathies, cardiomyopathies, electrolyte imbalances, and drug effects. Ventricular fibrillation occurs when the ventricular myocardium depolarizes erratically in an uncoordinated manner and shows fibrillation waves of varying amplitude and shape. There are no identifiable P waves, QRS complexes, or T waves, with a heart rate that can vary between 150 and 500 bpm. By definition, ventricular fibrillation is always unstable.[27] Signs and symptoms include but are not limited to palpitations (in chest or neck), chest pain, shortness of breath, generalized weakness, dizziness, diaphoresis, nausea, vomiting, syncope, or sudden death.

CORONARY ARTERY DISEASE

Atherosclerotic coronary artery disease (ASCAD) is the most common cause of death in athletes aged older than 35 years. It does still occur in a small percentage of young athletes as well, especially in those with inherited hyperlipidemia. For many, SCA is the first presenting symptom of ASCAD because acute events are caused by coronary plaque disruption and acute thrombosis rather than a gradual narrowing of coronary arteries. Vigorous exercise during competition will transiently increase the risk of acute myocardial infarction and SCA. This occurs by either an increased risk of plaque disruption or a malignant arrhythmia. Arrhythmias can develop from demand ischemia or can originate in an area of myocardial scarring. The risk of an acute exertion-related cardiac event is highest in those who have had earlier acute coronary syndrome and lower in those with "silent" ASCAD (found only through advanced/provocative diagnostic testing). The risk of SCA also increases with the extent of CAD, with lower left ventricular (LV) systolic function, with greater ischemia, and with increased electrical instability. The risk can be mitigated to some extent through aggressive lipid-lowering therapy, which can lower the lipid content of lipid-rich unstable plaques. This plaque regression can take as long as 2 years, and athletes with known ASCAD should exercise caution when deciding on their level of athletic competition.[28]

AORTIC DISSECTION OR RUPTURE (MARFAN SYNDROME)

Aortic pathologic condition in athletes is a common cause of sudden death in athletes due to the aortic stress that can occur during intense physical activity. Multiple predisposing aortic conditions besides Marfan syndrome can result in aortic dissection or rupture: familial thoracic aortic aneurysm, bicuspid aotic valve, aortic aneurysm, Loeys-Dietz syndrome. Marfan syndrome is an autosomal dominant disorder that affects connective tissue across multiple systems including the cardiac, pulmonary, musculoskeletal, skin, and ocular systems. The predominant gene mutation is in *fibrillin-1* and the incidence of disease is 1 in 5000 to 10,000.[29] Diagnosis of Marfan syndrome in adults relies on the Ghent criteria. Progressive aortic dilation with eventual aortic valve dysfunction can lead to aortic dissection, a tearing of the intima layer of the aorta, in athletes with Marfan syndrome.[30] Although it is known that mild aortic enlargement can occur from repetitive intense physical activity, aortic root dilation greater than 4 cm is abnormal and presents a risk for dissection. However, up to 12% of patients with Marfan and aortic dilation less than 4 cm still had an acute type A dissection.[31] Athletes with Marfan syndrome are recommended to participate in low and moderate static/low dynamic competitive sports if they do not meet exclusion criteria such as aortic root dilatation, moderate-to-severe mitral regurgitation, ejection fraction less than 40%, or a family history of aortic dissection at an aortic diameter of less than 5 cm.[29]

Sudden severe chest or upper back pain that may radiate to back or have a tearing or ripping sensation. Sudden severe abdominal pain, shortness of breath, sudden onset of neurologic symptoms, greater than 20 mm Hg difference in blood pressure between left and right arms or weaker pulses in one arm, decreased pulse strength, hypertension (more common), hypotension (sign of severe disease), tachycardia, syncope, or sudden death.

COMMOTIO CORDIS

Commotio cordis is ventricular fibrillation caused directly by blunt trauma to the heart, with no structural damage to the heart itself or surrounding structures. The mechanical distortion of the myocardium from the trauma creates enough mechanical energy to cause inappropriate cardiac depolarization, resulting in an unstable arrhythmia and cardiac arrest. It most commonly results from direct impact with a hard ball, such as a baseball. The impact must occur directly over the heart in the anterior chest during ventricular repolarization, during the upstroke just before the peak of the T wave. This occurs during about 1% of the cardiac cycle, although that can be higher with increased heart rates during exercise. The force from the impact causes a stretch in myocardial cell membranes, which may activate ion channels, specifically the stretch-sensitive K + $_{ATP}$ channel, leading to depolarization and ventricular fibrillation. The estimated energy required is approximately 50 J, and the risk peaks at around 40 mph for a baseball, as higher speeds are more likely to result in structural damage to the heart or chest wall. The risk of commotio cordis is also higher with smaller objects, and highest when the impact occurs over the center of the left ventricle. The risk can be reduced by softening the impact object or with chest protection, although studies have found that standard chest protectors are not designed to prevent commotio cordis, and do not prevent VF induction in laboratory experiments.[32]

ENVIRONMENTAL

Lightning strikes cause cardiac injury and sudden death through several pathways. Lightning delivers a current during the course of 0.001 to 0.1 seconds that can vary from 30,000 to 100,000 A.[12,33] This energy may pass over the surface of the victim or may penetrate to cause internal injuries. When the heart is involved, the energy from a lightning strike can cause cardiac contusion and pericardial disease, myocardial ischemia/infarction, myocardial stunning, arrhythmias, and aortic injury, including dissection.[33] Arrhythmias can be caused by the sudden increase in voltage from the lightning strike, which can depolarize the entire myocardium. They can also originate from increased autonomic stimulation and the associated catecholamine surge, which have an additive effect on the rate and rhythm. Ventricular tachycardia and ventricular fibrillation are the most common initial rhythms, although asystole is also frequently seen and may be caused primarily or secondary by medullary dysfunction. Nonfatal changes such as atrial fibrillation and QT prolongation have also been observed, possibly related to changes in intracellular calcium metabolism.[12] Cardiac contusion and aortic dissections can occur as a direct result of current passing through the myocardium or can be caused secondarily by explosive environmental effects leading to blunt or blast trauma. Patients with cardiac contusion can develop cardiac stunning and cardiogenic shock and can suffer morbidity and mortality up to several days after the initial strike. Cardiomyopathy may also develop, leading to cardiovascular compromise and ventricular failure. Pericarditis can also be a delayed response to a lightning strike, with myocardial inflammation and necrosis leading to pericardial effusions weeks to months afterward.[33]

EMERGENCY ACTION PLAN

The EAP is essential to proper cardiac emergency preparedness on the sideline. Development and review of the EAP should include proper communication techniques, emergency equipment location and training, integration of emergency responders, hospital transportation coordination, and catastrophic event training and preparedness. The EAP should be reviewed on an annual basis, at a minimum, with all stakeholders.

In the event of an unresponsive athlete, clear communication pathways should be designated in the EAP. We suggest the practice of nonverbal communication such as predetermined hand gestures to avoid difficulty in sending and receiving verbal communication in high volume settings such as a crowded stadium. However, the use of a primary and secondary backup verbal communication network such as walkie-talkie, cellphone, or satellite phone is recommended to allow for proper communication not only with on-site personnel but with hospital personnel as well. In large events or in remote areas, networks may be overloaded or unavailable, making equipment such as a satellite phone or landline particularly useful.

The location and availability of emergency equipment that include an AED will vary depending on the venue. However, the equipment should be placed in an easily accessible site that is not behind a locked door or gate. The location(s) should be a part of the EAP review. Emergency responder training in the use of an AED regardless of background is of the utmost importance. These responders can include school staff, students, teammates, team staff (eg, athletic trainer), EMS, or physicians. Equipment including AEDs should be checked during the annual review to ensure that they are still operational. AED battery life on standby, depending on the manufacturer, may last from 2 to 5 years in total. In the event an AED is used, the disposable pads should be replaced with a new set before being stored.

The level of expertise and involvement of EMS varies depending on the venue. The EAP should determine if EMS is on-site and off-site, what type of transportation is available, how they will be activated, and what level of technician is present. The levels of an emergency medical technician (EMT) across the different states in the United States may vary but typically are basic, intermediate, and advanced/paramedic. The EMT level will determine their capabilities and what type of equipment/medications they will have available. Coordination with EMS and the properly resourced receiving hospital is paramount in the successful resuscitation of an unresponsive athlete. The location of transportation, time and ease of access, and capabilities of the potential receiving hospitals should be listed in the EAP.

The level of preparedness of every EAP-listed emergency responder will determine the success of a cardiac resuscitation. A well-run resuscitation should be efficient, smooth, quiet, and without much wasted effort. Preassignment of duties, including a team leader, should be detailed in the EAP.

In the unfortunate circumstance of a cardiac resuscitation, a postevent protocol should be detailed in the EAP. The event should be documented, analyzed, debriefed, and used for quality improvement. Administrative, legal, and emotional support should be activated for involved parties.

GENERAL PREPARTICIPATION PHYSICAL EXAMINATION CONSIDERATIONS

A detailed history of the athlete's symptoms during and outside of exercise remains one of the most important tools in the preparticipation cardiac screening evaluation. Care should be taken to ask about any chest pain or chest pain equivalents, shortness of breath, fevers, chills, history of syncope—exertional or otherwise, family history of sudden death or cardiac disease.

The physical examination should focus on findings associated with conditions that might predispose an athlete to sudden cardiac arrest. The most common findings on examination that would prompt further workup include heart murmur, especially a systolic murmur that increases with Valsalva, Marfanoid features (long, narrow face, tall, thin body build, disproportionately long arms, legs, fingers, and toes, abnormal spine or sternum curvature, extreme nearsightedness, flat feet), or abnormal rhythm or resting tachycardia/bradycardia.

There is considerable debate about the cost-effectiveness and appropriateness of diagnostic testing as a part of routine preparticipation physical exam (PPE) screening, which is outside the scope of this article. When further workup is indicated, however, cardiac testing may include ECG, echocardiogram, stress test, or cardiac MRI.

EVALUATION OF OUTCOME AND/OR LONG-TERM RECOMMENDATIONS

Athletes who suffer cardiac arrest events who achieve ROSC and are subsequently stabilized will need extensive postarrest care. Initial steps should include emergent transport to the nearest appropriate hospital for intensive care unit (ICU) admission and specialty Cardiology evaluation. The underlying cause of the arrest will determine what further treatment modalities are required. Patients who suffer an arrest secondary to an arrhythmia should have testing including electrocardiogram, echocardiogram, and an electrophysiological study to help determine the underlying cause of the arrest. These patients generally need an implantable defibrillator because patients who have suffered a cardiac arrest are at a much higher risk for repeat arrhythmia/arrest. Patients who also have an underlying cardiomyopathy may need symptomatic treatment as well as preventative measures to avoid future events. Those with hypertrophic cardiomyopathy that results in outflow tract obstruction may benefit from heart failure medications such as beta-blockers, calcium-channel blockers, or diuretics. HCM patients with marked outflow obstruction unresponsive to medical therapy may also be candidates for ventricular septal surgical myectomy or alcohol septal ablation.[34] ARVC patients will typically need similar treatment of heart failure symptoms related to their cardiomyopathy, with medical management, lifestyle changes, and catheter ablation.[35] Patients with cardiomyopathy not adequately responsive to these treatments may ultimately progress to a need for heart transplantation. Recommendations for patients with a definitive diagnosis of HCM or ARVC include restriction from competitive and high-intensity sports, and possible restriction from low-intensity recreational sports and athletic activities, depending on their individual risk.[34] Patients suffering a cardiac arrest following a commotio cordis event should undergo testing for underlying structural heart abnormalities but may be able to fully return to play if the heart is normal and the athlete has no other long-term effects. See **Fig. 1** for recommended management guidelines for HCM.

CORONARY ARTERY DISEASE

Athletes with ASCAD should undergo exercise testing to determine the presence and extent of inducible ischemia and electrical instability as well as to evaluate LV function. They should have aggressive statin therapy to reduce the risk of plaque disruption and must weigh the risks and benefits of exercise when determining level of future competition. Athletes with LV ejection fraction greater than 50% and no inducible ischemia or electrical instability should be allowed to participate in all levels of competition. It is reasonable to restrict athletes with a higher disease burden, and athletes who have an AMI or who undergo coronary revascularization should refrain from competitive sports for at least 3 months.[28]

MYOCARDITIS

Athletes with suspected myocarditis should have diagnostics that include an ECG, cardiac biomarkers (troponin, natriuretic peptide, creatine kinase), inflammatory markers, chest radiograph, and echocardiogram. In suspected COVID-19 infection, a COVID-19 polymerase chain reaction test (PCR) should be performed as well. The gold standard for noninvasive diagnostics is cardiac MRI (cMR), whereas an

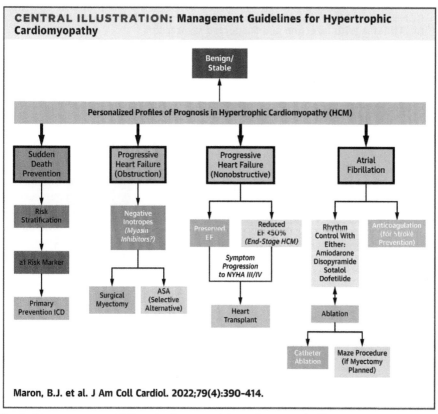

Fig. 1. Management guidelines for hypertrophic cardiomyopathy.[34]

endomyocardial biopsy is the invasive standard. In cases where the cMR is inconclusive, a fluorodeoxyglucose positron emission tomography scan can be considered.[36] Although there are multiple diagnostic modalities to evaluate for myocarditis, to date, there are no universally accepted diagnostic clinical criteria for myocarditis. However, Eichhorn and colleagues have suggested a diagnostic pathway for athletes that uses ECG, Holter monitor, stress test, cardiac biomarkers, inflammatory biomarkers, or echocardiogram as a screening tool.[19] Refer to **Fig. 2** for their proposed diagnostic and treatment algorithm for myocarditis. If one of these tests is positive, cMR is used to investigate for evidence of myocarditis. If a diagnosis of myocarditis is made, exercise and sports restriction is recommended for a minimum of 3 months. After symptoms have resolved, repeat testing with echocardiogram, Holter monitoring, and possible cMR is recommended at 3 months. If symptoms have not resolved, reevaluation every 3 months is recommended.[37]

DISSECTION

Long-term management of aortic dissection includes close regulation of blood pressure and heart rate. In athletes who survive an aortic dissection, care must be taken to minimize the risk of worsening the dissection through rupture or recurrent dissection, which can happen through increased aortic wall shear stress. This increased

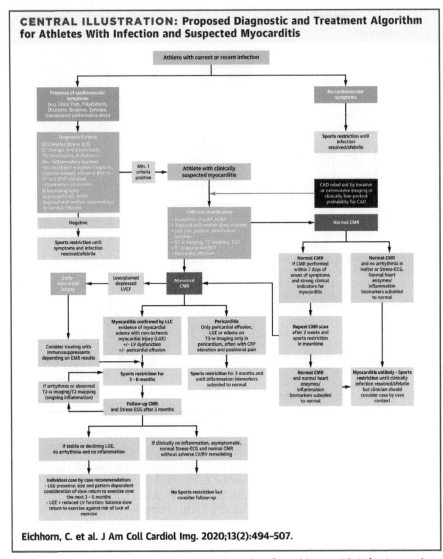

Fig. 2. Proposed diagnostic and treatment algorithm for athletes with infection and suspected myocarditis.[19]

stress can occur with sudden increases in arterial blood pressure and heart rate, such as during exercise, and is most significant in higher intensity activities such as weight-lifting or running. However, maintaining regular exercise can still be a benefit to these patients in terms of reaching long-term blood pressure, heart rate, and body weight goals. Recommendations generally advise that mild-to-moderate intensity aerobic exercise (3–5 metabolic equivalents) for at least 30 minutes a day is beneficial. Weight-lifting should be limited to lighter weights and athletes should stop several repetitions before failure to avoid straining. Higher intensity exercises and competition should generally be avoided.[38,39] In patients with Marfan syndrome, varying organizations have created specific activity recommendations (**Fig. 3**).[40]

Current Sport /Exercise Recommendations For Patients with MFS or Other Aortic Conditions

Society / Organization	Recommendations
COMPETETIVE ATHLETES	
Bethesda Guidelines (2005) for MFS	• May participate in low and moderate static / low dynamic competitive sports if they do not have the following: ❖ Aortic root dilation >4.0cm in adults, or 2SD from the mean for BSA in children ❖ Moderate-to-severe MR ❖ Family history of dissection of SCD in a Marfan relative • Athletes should repeat echo measurement of aorta every 6 months
ESC Guidelines (2005) for MFS	• No competitive sports
NON-COMETETIVE ATHLETES	
AHA Scientific Statement for MFS	• No burst activities (rapid acceleration / deceleration) • Avoid intense isometric activities • Avoid extreme environmental conditions or extreme sports (bungee jumping / hang gliding) • Avoid collision sports
AHA/ACC Aortic Guidelines (2010)	• Avoid collision sports and strenuous activities involving lifting, pushing, or straining that require Valsalva for individuals with thoracic aortic disease
ESC Aortic Guidelines (2014)	• Avoid isometric exercise with a high static load in anyone with an elastopathy or BAV with a dilated root (>4.0cm)
The Marfan Foundation	• Favor non-competitive, dynamic exercises such as brisk walking, jogging, leisurely bicycling or slow-paced tennis • During exercise maintain a HR <110 or <100 if on B-blockers • Avoid isometric activities (push-up / sit-ups/ weightlifting) • Avoid contact sports
Loeys-Dietz Foundation	• Avoid competitive sports, especially contact sports, or muscle straining activities performed to the point of exhaustion. • Avoid straining activities such as push-ups, chin-ups, sit-ups • Remain active with aerobic types of activities that are performed at moderate aerobic hiking, biking, jogging, swimming

Recreational (Non-competitive) Sports & Exercise Recommendations in Marfan Patients (Assumes no or minimal aortic dilation)

Permitted	Intermediate[a]	Strongly Discouraged
• Bowling • Golf • Brisk Walking • Modest Hiking • Tennis (Doubles) • Treadmill • Stationary bike	• Basketball • Touch football • Tennis (single) • Skiing (Downhill or cross country) • Running • Soccer • Hiking • Swimming (lap) • Horseback riding • Biking	• Body building • Ice hockey • Rock climbing • Windsurfing • Surfing • Scuba diving • Weightlifting (free weights)

Fig. 3. Physical activity recommendations for athletes with Marfan syndrome from varying organizations.[a]Intermediate or indeterminate activities should be assessed clinically on an individual basis.

SICKLE CELL TRAIT

Although SCT is not a contraindication to participation in athletics, screening for sickle cell trait during PPEs is of the utmost importance. If SCT status is unknown, a hemoglobin solubility test and subsequent hemoglobin electrophoresis can help to identify HgbS and its subtypes, respectively.

Return to play should not be considered until the athlete is asymptomatic at rest and has normal end-organ function. Bloodwork such as a complete blood count, comprehensive metabolic panel, creatine kinase, lactate dehydrogenase, uric acid, and disseminated intravascular coagulation panel should be resolved to baseline. Assessment of identifiable event risk factors or uncovered risk factors such as hydration status, heat, altitude, pharmaceutical influence (eg, sympathomimetic, caffeine, other stimulants, and so forth.), abnormal work–rest ratio, poor electrolyte supplementation, chronic kidney disease, evidence of hyposthenuria, or other genetic anomaly will influence the decision for the athlete to return to play.[11]

A schedule to allow for gradual conditioning, exclusion from performance tests, an emphasis on hydration and electrolyte replacement, modifications for an athlete at altitude with supplemental oxygen if needed, and careful observation for concomitant acute illnesses can help prevent sickle collapse. However, despite these methods, sickle collapse can still occur.[24]

CORONARY ARTERY ANOMALIES

Long-term recommendations after diagnosis of CAA are athlete-dependent but there are generalizable recommendations. The athlete must have confirmatory imaging, a negative exercise stress test, and be asymptomatic.[23] If the athlete has surgical repair of an anomalous aortic origin of a coronary artery, the minimum time before participation is at least 3 months postoperative. The athlete must be asymptomatic and must not demonstrate ischemia on a maximal exercise stress test. Overall, as demonstrated in **Table 1**, recommendations are highly variable and depend on the specific anomaly in question.

SUMMARY/DISCUSSION/FUTURE DIRECTIONS

A moment of tragedy can be prevented and reversed with proper preparedness through a careful PPE and practiced EAP. The approach and management to SCD are the same despite multiple causes. Although the medical community has made great strides in standardizing CPR response, more evidence-based guidance should be developed for the at-risk or returning athlete.

Table 1
A comparison of current international guidelines for exercise restrictions in patients with coronary artery anomalies

Comparison of Current International Guidelines for Exercise Restrictions in Patients With CAAs

2015 ACC/AHA scientific statement for competitive athletes with cardiovascular abnormalities			2020 ESC guidelines on sports cardiology and exercise in patients with cardiovascular disease		
COR	LOE	Recommendations	COR	LOE	Recommendations
			IIa	C	When considering sports activities, evaluation with imaging tests to identify high-risk patterns and an exercise stress test to check for ischemia should be considered in individuals with AAOC.
			IIb	C	In asymptomatic individuals with an anomalous coronary artery that does not course between the large vessels or does not have a slit-like orifice with reduced lumen or intramural course, competition may be considered after adequate counseling on the risks provided that there is an absence of inducible ischemia.
			III	C	Participation in most competitive sports with a moderate or high cardiovascular demand among individuals with AAOC with an acutely angled takeoff or an anomalous course between the large vessels is not recommended.*
IIa	C	Athletes with AAORCA should be evaluated by an exercise stress test. For those without either symptoms or a positive exercise stress test, permission to compete can be considered after adequate counseling of the athlete or the athlete's parents (in the case of a minor) about the risk and benefit, taking into consideration the uncertainty of the accuracy of a negative stress test.			
III	B	Athletes with AAOLCA, especially when the artery passes between the pulmonary artery and aorta, should be restricted from participation in all competitive sports, with the possible exception of class IA sports, before surgical repair. This recommendation applies whether the anomaly is identified as a consequence of symptoms or discovered incidentally.			
III	C	Nonoperated athletes with AAORCA who exhibit symptoms, arrhythmias, or signs of ischemia on exercise stress test should be restricted from participation in all competitive sports, with the possible exception of class IA sports, before a surgical repair.			
IIb	C	After successful surgical repair of AAOC, athletes may consider participation in all sports 3 mo after surgery if the patient remains free of symptoms and an exercise stress test shows no evidence of ischemia or cardiac arrhythmias.	IIb	C	After surgical repair of an AAOC, participation in all sports may be considered, at the earliest 3 mo after surgery, if the athletes are asymptomatic and there is no evidence of inducible myocardial ischemia or complex cardiac arrhythmias during maximal exercise stress test.
I	C	Athletes with APOC artery can participate only in low-intensity class IA sports, regardless of whether they have had a prior myocardial infarction, and pending repair of the anomaly.			
IIb	C	After repair of APOC, decisions about exercise restriction may be based on presence of sequelae such as myocardial infarction or ventricular dysfunction.			
IIa	C	It is reasonable for athletes with myocardial bridging and no evidence of myocardial ischemia during adequate stress testing to participate in all competitive sports.	IIa	C	Participation in competitive and leisure-time sports should be considered in asymptomatic individuals with myocardial bridging and without inducible ischemia or ventricular arrhythmia during maximal exercise testing.
IIa	C	It is reasonable to restrict athletes with myocardial bridging of an epicardial coronary artery and objective evidence of myocardial ischemia or prior myocardial infarction to sports with low to moderate dynamic and low to moderate static demands.	III	C	Competitive sports are not recommended in individuals with myocardial bridging and persistent ischemia or complex cardiac arrhythmias during maximal exercise stress testing.
IIa	C	It is reasonable to restrict athletes who have undergone surgical resection of the myocardial bridge or stenting of the bridge to low-intensity sports for 6 mo after the procedure. If such athletes have no subsequent evidence of ischemia, they may participate in all competitive sports.			

CLINICS CARE POINTS

- Cardiac emergencies are a significant cause of morbidity and mortality in athletes and are the leading nontraumatic cause of death in the young athlete.
- Prompt evaluation and treatment of the collapsed athlete are vital to maximizing their chances of survival.
- Formal planning for an efficient and effective response care can help avoid catastrophic outcomes.
- Initial management of cardiac emergencies includes the activation of EMS, early CPR, rapid defibrillation, and transfer to an appropriate medical center.
- Sudden cardiac arrest should be suspected in any collapsed and unresponsive athlete, and an AED should be used as early as possible, with CPR taking place until it can be applied.
- Interruptions in chest compressions for rhythm analysis and defibrillation should be minimized, and compressions should resume immediately after a shock is delivered.
- Underlying cardiac abnormalities that can predispose some athletes to sudden cardiac arrest include cardiomyopathies, CAAs, and channelopathies, as well as genetic disorders such as sickle cell trait, and Marfan syndrome.
- Screening for cardiac abnormalities is an important strategy in trying to prevent sudden cardiac arrest, although the sensitivity, specificity, and cost-effectiveness of the current screening practices are ongoing topics of debate.
- Cardiac arrest secondary to commotio cordis should be suspected in any athlete who collapses shortly after being struck in the chest.
- Lightning strikes are a rare but potentially fatal cause of cardiac emergencies and can cause both short-term and long-term injuries to the patient's heart.

DISCLOSURE

No commercial or financial conflicts of interest or funding sources for either author.

REFERENCES

1. Harmon KG, Asif IM, Maleszewski JJ, et al. Incidence, cause, and comparative frequency of sudden cardiac death in national collegiate athletic association athletes a decade in review. Circulation 2015;132(1). https://doi.org/10.1161/CIRCULATIONAHA.115.015431.
2. Paratz ED, Smith K, Ball J, et al. The economic impact of sudden cardiac arrest. Resuscitation 2021;163. https://doi.org/10.1016/j.resuscitation.2021.04.001.
3. Valenzuela TD, Roe DJ, Nichol G, et al. Outcomes of Rapid Defibrillation by Security Officers after Cardiac Arrest in Casinos. N Engl J Med 2000;343(17). https://doi.org/10.1056/nejm200010263431701.
4. Larsen MP, Eisenberg MS, Cummins RO, et al. Predicting survival from out-of-hospital cardiac arrest: A graphic model. Ann Emerg Med 1993;22(11). https://doi.org/10.1016/S0196-0644(05)81302-2.
5. Park GJ, Song KJ, Shin S Do, et al. Timely bystander CPR improves outcomes despite longer EMS times. Am J Emerg Med 2017;35(8). https://doi.org/10.1016/j.ajem.2017.02.033.
6. Hazinski MF, Nolan JP, Aickin R, et al. Part 1: Executive summary: 2015 International consensus on cardiopulmonary resuscitation and emergency cardiovascular care

science with treatment recommendations. Circulation 2015;132. https://doi.org/10.1161/CIR.0000000000000270.

7. Kleinman ME, Brennan EE, Goldberger ZD, et al. Part 5: Adult basic life support and cardiopulmonary resuscitation quality: 2015 American Heart Association guidelines update for cardiopulmonary resuscitation and emergency cardiovascular care. Circulation 2015;132(18). https://doi.org/10.1161/CIR.0000000000000259.

8. Bobrow BJ, Spaite DW, Berg RA, et al. Chest compression-only CPR by lay rescuers and survival from out-of-hospital cardiac arrest. JAMA 2010;304(13). https://doi.org/10.1001/jama.2010.1392.

9. Yılmaz G, Bol O. Comparison of femoral and carotid arteries in terms of pulse check in cardiopulmonary resuscitation: A prospective observational study. Resuscitation 2021;162. https://doi.org/10.1016/j.resuscitation.2021.01.042.

10. West RL, Otto Q, Drennan IR, et al. CPR-related cognitive activity, consciousness, awareness and recall, and its management: A scoping review. Resusc Plus 2022; 10:100241.

11. O'Connor FG, Franzos MA, Nye NS, et al. Summit on Exercise Collapse Associated with Sickle Cell Trait: Finding the "way Ahead. Curr Sports Med Rep 2021; 20(1). https://doi.org/10.1249/JSR.0000000000000801.

12. van Ruler R, Eikendal T, Kooij FO, et al. A shocking injury: A clinical review of lightning injuries highlighting pitfalls and a treatment protocol. Injury 2022; 53(10):3070–7.

13. Marian AJ, Braunwald E. Hypertrophic cardiomyopathy: Genetics, pathogenesis, clinical manifestations, diagnosis, and therapy. Circ Res 2017;121(7). https://doi.org/10.1161/CIRCRESAHA.117.311059.

14. Corrado D, Basso C. Arrhythmogenic left ventricular cardiomyopathy. Heart 2022;108(9):733–43.

15. Zecchin M, Muser D, Vitali-Serdoz L, et al. Arrhythmias in Dilated Cardiomyopathy: Diagnosis and Treatment. In: Dilated cardiomyopathy. ; 2019. https://doi.org/10.1007/978-3-030-13864-6_10.

16. Tse G, Liu T, Li KHC, et al. Electrophysiological mechanisms of Brugada syndrome: Insights from pre-clinical and clinical studies. Front Physiol 2016; 7(OCT). https://doi.org/10.3389/fphys.2016.00467.

17. Johannes S, Jürgen B, Christoph B, et al. Diagnosis, risk stratification and treatment of Brugada syndrome. Dtsch Arztebl Int 2015;112(23). https://doi.org/10.3238/arztebl.2015.0394.

18. Li KHC, Lee S, Yin C, et al. Brugada syndrome: A comprehensive review of pathophysiological mechanisms and risk stratification strategies. IJC Hear Vasc 2020; 26:100468.

19. Eichhorn C, Bière L, Schnell F, et al. Myocarditis in Athletes Is a Challenge: Diagnosis, Risk Stratification, and Uncertainties. JACC Cardiovasc Imaging 2020; 13(2). https://doi.org/10.1016/j.jcmg.2019.01.039.

20. Halle M, Binzenhöfer L, Mahrholdt H, et al. Myocarditis in athletes: A clinical perspective. Eur J Prev Cardiol 2021;28(10). https://doi.org/10.1177/2047487320909670.

21. Modica G, Bianco M, Sollazzo F, et al. Myocarditis in Athletes Recovering from COVID-19: A Systematic Review and Meta-Analysis. Int J Environ Res Public Health 2022;19(7):4279.

22. Villa AD, Sammut E, Nair A, et al. Coronary artery anomalies overview: The normal and the abnormal. World J Radiol 2016;8(6). https://doi.org/10.4329/wjr.v8.i6.537.

23. Gentile F, Castiglione V, De Caterina R. Coronary Artery Anomalies. Circulation 2021;144:983–96.

24. Harmon KG, Drezner JA, Klossner D, et al. Sickle cell trait associated with a RR of death of 37 times in national collegiate athletic association football athletes: A database with 2 million athlete-years as the denominator. Br J Sports Med 2012;46(5). https://doi.org/10.1136/bjsports-2011-090896.
25. Maron BJ, Harris KM, Thompson PD, et al. Eligibility and Disqualification Recommendations for Competitive Athletes With Cardiovascular Abnormalities: Task Force 14: Sickle Cell Trait. J Am Coll Cardiol 2015;66(21). https://doi.org/10.1016/j.jacc.2015.09.046.
26. Tsaras G, Owusu-Ansah A, Boateng FO, et al. Complications Associated with Sickle Cell Trait: A Brief Narrative Review. Am J Med 2009;122(6):507–12.
27. Enriquez A, Frankel DS, Baranchuk A. Pathophysiology of ventricular tachyarrhythmias: From automaticity to reentry. Herzschrittmachertherap Elektrophysiol 2017;28(2). https://doi.org/10.1007/s00399-017-0512-4.
28. Thompson PD, Myerburg RJ, Levine BD, et al. Eligibility and Disqualification Recommendations for Competitive Athletes With Cardiovascular Abnormalities: Task Force 8: Coronary Artery Disease. J Am Coll Cardiol 2015;66(21). https://doi.org/10.1016/j.jacc.2015.09.040.
29. Braverman AC, Harris KM, Kovacs RJ, et al. Eligibility and Disqualification Recommendations for Competitive Athletes With Cardiovascular Abnormalities: Task Force 7: Aortic Diseases, Including Marfan Syndrome. J Am Coll Cardiol 2015;66(21). https://doi.org/10.1016/j.jacc.2015.09.039.
30. Dean JCS. Marfan syndrome: Clinical diagnosis and management. Eur J Hum Genet 2007;15(7). https://doi.org/10.1038/sj.ejhg.5201851.
31. Parish LM, Gorman JH, Kahn S, et al. Aortic size in acute type A dissection: implications for preventive ascending aortic replacement. Eur J Cardio-thoracic Surg. 2009;35(6). https://doi.org/10.1016/j.ejcts.2008.12.047.
32. Link MS. Pathophysiology, prevention, and treatment of commotio cordis. Curr Cardiol Rep 2014;16(6). https://doi.org/10.1007/s11886-014-0495-2.
33. Christophides T, Khan S, Ahmad M, et al. Cardiac Effects of Lightning Strikes. Arrhythmia Electrophysiol Rev 2017;6(3):114.
34. Maron BJ, Desai MY, Nishimura RA, et al. Management of Hypertrophic Cardiomyopathy: JACC State-of-the-Art Review. J Am Coll Cardiol 2022;79(4). https://doi.org/10.1016/j.jacc.2021.11.021.
35. Corrado D, Wichter T, Link MS, et al. Treatment of arrhythmogenic right ventricular cardiomyopathy/dysplasia: An international task force consensus statement. Eur Heart J 2015;36(46). https://doi.org/10.1093/eurheartj/ehv162.
36. Lampejo T, Durkin SM, Bhatt N, et al. Acute myocarditis: Aetiology, diagnosis and management. Clin Med J R Coll Physicians London 2021;21(5). https://doi.org/10.7861/clinmed.2021-0121.
37. Hurwitz B, Issa O. Management and Treatment of Myocarditis in Athletes. Curr Treat Options Cardiovasc Med 2020;22(12). https://doi.org/10.1007/s11936-020-00875-1.
38. Spanos K, Tsilimparis N, Kölbel T. Exercise after Aortic Dissection: to Run or Not to Run. Eur J Vasc Endovasc Surg 2018;55(6). https://doi.org/10.1016/j.ejvs.2018.03.009.
39. Chaddha A, Eagle KA, Braverman AC, et al. Exercise and physical activity for the post-aortic dissection patient: The clinician's conundrum. Clin Cardiol 2015;38(11). https://doi.org/10.1002/clc.22481.
40. Cheng A, Owens D. Marfan syndrome, inherited aortopathies and exercise: What is the right answer? Br J Sports Med 2016;50(2):100–4.

Acute Emergent Airway Issues in Sports

Mary Terese Whipple, MD[a,b,*], Jeffrey P. Feden, MD[c]

KEYWORDS

- Sideline • Airway • Emergency • Sports medicine • Airway assessment
- Airway intervention

KEY POINTS

- The initial approach to airway management and intervention focuses on the assessment of three basic considerations: failure to oxygenate, failure to ventilate, and failure to maintain airway patency.
- Airway obstruction is immediately life-threatening and may result from many different causes. Prompt recognition and intervention are necessary to relieve the obstruction and restore oxygenation and ventilation.
- The differential diagnosis for airway emergency can be divided into several classes to aid in identifying the etiology of respiratory distress or airway compromise: obtundation/apnea, upper airway compromise, and lower airway compromise.
- A simple airway positioning maneuver is often sufficient to establish airway patency in an unconscious athlete. The two most common methods for opening the airway are the head-tilt/chin-lift and jaw-thrust maneuvers.
- Various airway adjuncts can be used if airway repositioning fails including an oropharyngeal airway, nasopharyngeal airway, and supraglottic devices. If these fail, intubation or a surgical airway may be necessary.

INTRODUCTION

Although rarely encountered in sports medicine practice, there are few scenarios that are more pressing than an airway emergency or impending airway compromise in an athlete. The well-known "ABC" mnemonic refers to the sequence of functions that are vital to life—airway, breathing, and circulation—and must be considered for intervention when encountering an ill or injured person. Only chest compressions and early

[a] Department of Emergency Medicine, University of Iowa Hospitals and Clinics, 200 Hawkins Drive, 1008 RCP, Iowa City, IA 52246, USA; [b] Department of Orthopedics and Rehabilitation, University of Iowa Hospitals and Clinics, 200 Hawkins Drive, 1008 RCP, Iowa City, IA 52246, USA; [c] Department of Emergency Medicine, Alpert Medical School of Brown University, 593 Eddy Street, Davol 141, Providence, RI 02903, USA
* Corresponding author.
E-mail address: mary-whipple@uiowa.edu
Twitter: @Twhip21 (M.T.W.)

Clin Sports Med 42 (2023) 373–384
https://doi.org/10.1016/j.csm.2023.02.004
0278-5919/23/© 2023 Elsevier Inc. All rights reserved.

defibrillation in the case of cardiac arrest will take priority over airway management. Therefore, an understanding of rapid airway assessment and basic airway maneuvers is critical for sports medicine practitioners. More advanced airway management techniques and equipment may be utilized by those with proper training and experience but may still present challenges in the prehospital setting.

AIRWAY ASSESSMENT

The initial approach to airway management and intervention focuses on the assessment of three basic considerations: failure to oxygenate, failure to ventilate, and failure to maintain airway patency. Airway emergencies may present with any or a combination of these concerns. The proper technique for airway management is then determined by the cause of airway compromise and condition of the athlete and may include invasive and/or noninvasive measures.

Evaluation for airway obstruction is the essential first step in assessment, and level of consciousness can be an important indicator of airway patency. An awake and conscious athlete with the ability to speak is presumed to have a patent airway at that moment. The unconscious athlete, however, should be considered to have airway obstruction until proven otherwise. Complete airway obstruction is immediately life-threatening and may result from foreign body aspiration, trauma, anaphylaxis, or even blockage of the hypopharynx by the tongue. Prompt recognition and intervention are necessary to relieve the obstruction and restore oxygenation and ventilation. Complete obstruction may present with acute distress, obtundation, or cardiopulmonary arrest. Interventions range from simple maneuvers to open the airway (eg, head-tilt-chin-lift, jaw-thrust) to the use of adjunctive devices, tracheal intubation, or cricothyrotomy. Partial airway obstruction is characterized by findings such as anxiety, altered mental status, labored breathing or respiratory distress, or airway noises such as stridor.

Although an obstructed airway will be rapidly fatal due to absent or impaired air exchange, the inability to oxygenate or ventilate can still occur in the setting of airway patency and should also be considered in the airway assessment. Hypoxia and hypoventilation can present with dyspnea, tachypnea, increased work of breathing, accessory muscle use, wheezing, cyanosis, agitation, and altered mental status. Interventions vary based on the underlying condition.

It is important to recognize the dynamic nature of airway compromise and the need for frequent re-assessment when airway concerns exist. Partial obstruction may progress to complete obstruction, and anticipation of an airway emergency in an initially well-appearing athlete should not be underestimated. Examples include anaphylaxis and neck trauma with progressive swelling or an expanding hematoma causing airway compression. Although airway interventions may not be immediately necessary, early activation of emergency medical services for transport to the emergency department must be strongly considered when the clinical circumstances warrant.

BASIC AIRWAY TECHNIQUES AND EQUIPMENT

Advanced airway management skills often require an experienced clinician, but basic airway maneuvers and equipment should be familiar to all. Following airway assessment, choosing the proper technique and/or device is the next step in airway management when intervention is indicated.

Facemask Removal

Helmeted athletes present a unique challenge to the sports medicine practitioner particularly when the helmet has an attached facemask. Airway access is a prerequisite to airway management. Facemask removal is a critical step that should occur in parallel with airway assessment. Given the wide variety of helmet styles and brands used in any particular sport, the technique and equipment used for removal of the facemask should be reviewed regularly.

Airway Positioning

A simple airway positioning maneuver is often sufficient to establish airway patency in an unconscious athlete. The two most common methods for opening the airway are the head-tilt/chin-lift and jaw-thrust maneuvers. Head-tilt/chin-lift is generally preferred but should be avoided if cervical spine immobilization is necessary. When there is concern for cervical spine injury, the jaw-thrust maneuver allows the tongue to be cleared from the airway without manipulating the cervical spine. The use of suction is another simple technique that can be effective in clearing secretions, such as blood and vomit, from the airway.

Airway Adjuncts

The oropharyngeal airway (OPA) and nasopharyngeal airway (NPA) are airway adjunctive devices that may be used to relieve upper airway obstruction. However, these devices will not be effective in treating supraglottic or other lower airway obstructions. OPAs and NPAs are available in different sizes and should be appropriately sized to the individual patient. The OPA is intended to open the airway by preventing the tongue from obstructing the posterior oropharynx, especially in the unconscious, supine patient. An OPA is contraindicated and will not be tolerated in patients with an intact gag reflex. It should also be avoided when airway obstruction is related to a foreign body as insertion of an OPA can force the foreign body further into the airway, worsening the obstruction. The NPA passes through the nostril into the posterior oropharynx, also serving to relieve anatomic obstruction similar to the OPA. However, the advantage of the NPA is that it does not stimulate the gag reflex and may, therefore, be an effective tool in the awake or semiconscious patient requiring basic airway support. NPAs are also useful adjuncts when the oral cavity cannot be easily accessed for reasons such as trismus or angioedema but should be avoided in cases of facial trauma. OPAs and NPAs are commonly used in conjunction with bag-valve-mask ventilation to establish airway patency for the delivery of oxygenation and ventilation. They are best applied as a temporizing measure until a reversible airway issue is resolved or as a bridge to advanced airway management in more complicated cases.

Bag Mask Ventilation

Ventilation using a bag-valve-mask (BVM) device is considered a basic life support technique but is, in reality, a difficult skill to master and requires practice. BVM ventilation requires an accompanying oxygen source and is often performed with airway positioning maneuvers in addition to an oropharyngeal or nasopharyngeal airway adjunct. Although effective BVM ventilation can be accomplished by a single operator, a second person dedicated to ensuring a proper mask seal generally allows for better technique. Indications for use of a BVM include the inability to oxygenate and/or ventilate. Airway obstruction not remedied by use of an OPA or NPA will render BVM ventilation ineffective.

Advanced Airway Techniques and Equipment

Advanced airway management, such as tracheal intubation, is unlikely to be undertaken in most sports medicine settings or by clinicians without proper training or experience. Athletic events that may be more commonly associated with high-energy trauma warrant emergency medical services personnel or other qualified health care providers who are skilled in advanced techniques. However, all sports medicine practitioners should be familiar with advanced airway equipment, such as supraglottic devices.

Supraglottic devices, such as the laryngeal mask airway and King tube, are often preferred to tracheal intubation in the prehospital setting because of their ease of use in securing an airway. Both can be placed blindly into the oropharynx to provide oxygenation and ventilation when connected to a self-inflating bag (ie, Ambu bag) and oxygen source. It should be noted that these devices are used neither for patients with a gag reflex nor to provide a definitive airway; rather, they are most commonly deployed in cases of cardiopulmonary arrest. In such cases, supraglottic devices are reliable alternatives for advanced airway management by inexperienced operators.[1]

Tracheal intubation is the gold standard for advanced airway management and allows for definitive control of the airway to enable effective gas exchange and prevent aspiration. Patients undergoing intubation must be sedated and paralyzed, and placement of the endotracheal tube is accomplished by visualization of the larynx (ie, direct laryngoscopy) or indirectly using other adjunctive devices such as a Bougie. A surgical airway, or cricothyrotomy, is a rescue technique in which a small incision is made to the anterior neck, and subsequently, the cricothyroid membrane allows passage of a tube directly into the trachea. Cricothyrotomy requires training and knowledge of the relevant anatomy. It is reserved as a last resort in cases of failed intubation or inability to access the airway for reasons including facial trauma or supraglottic obstruction.

Differential Diagnosis

The team physician should ask the athlete about the events leading up to the airway emergency, or if unconscious, the athletic trainer, coach, parent, or teammates. Questions about medical history, allergies, and current medication usage can be important for determining the etiology of the airway emergency and the best course of treatment. If the athlete is unconscious and there was a possibility of neck trauma, in-line cervical spine stabilization should be maintained.

The differential diagnosis for sideline airway emergencies is broad but can be organized into categories that make isolating the cause easier: airway issues due to altered level of consciousness and/or apnea, upper airway issues, and lower airway issues.

Level of Consciousness/Apnea

The obtunded athlete

The approach to airway management in an athlete with decreased level of consciousness is similar for most causes including significant head trauma, seizure, hypoglycemia, hyponatremia, and return of spontaneous circulation after cardiac arrest. Assessment proceeds according to basic life support (BLS) and advanced cardiovascular life support (ACLS) as previously outlined, first assessing the airway for patency, then breathing, and finally circulation. If the athlete can phonate, then the airway is patent. If the athlete is obtunded or unable to phonate, then secondary signs must be used to assess airway patency. Listen for evidence of snoring respirations and/or stridor indicating that the airway is blocked. Look for evidence of chest rise indicating spontaneous respirations and effective ventilation. In the case of cardiac arrest, the athlete may appear to be taking some spontaneous breaths, however, respirations may be agonal and ineffective for oxygenation and respiration and require intervention.

If snoring respirations are observed, or the athlete appears to be making some respiratory effort but without obvious air exchange or chest rise, then the airway should be repositioned to remove any obstruction. A head-tilt chin-lift maneuver can be attempted. However, if cervical spine stabilization is required, the head-tilt chin-lift maneuver can cause too much cervical spine motion. Instead, a jaw-thrust should be performed to pull the tongue forward and relieve its obstruction of the oropharynx. If a jaw-thrust does not improve air movement, then one of several airway adjuncts should be attempted as described previously including OPA, NPA, supraglottic airway, or intubation if the provider is skilled in this intervention.

Seizure

Traditionally, people with seizure disorders had been discouraged from participating in sports. However, over the last few decades, recommendations have changed and more and more athletes with epilepsy have been entering the sporting world.[2] As a result, sideline physicians should be well versed in first aid for seizures and management of the airway when a seizure does occur.

Seizures can be convulsive or non-convulsive. Non-convulsive seizures are unlikely to require airway intervention as the patient most often maintains their airway and breathing, although they may have an altered level of consciousness.

Tonic-clonic seizures may require basic airway support measures or even a definitive airway. Tonic-clonic seizures usually begin with a period of stiffening of the body (the tonic phase). During the tonic phase, the athlete may go apneic and be transiently hypoxic. However, this phase is usually short-lived, and respirations will resume once the clonic phase begins.[3] If possible, the athlete should be lowered gently to the ground and laid on their side to facilitate airway clearing. Apnea should be brief, however, if the patient does not resume breathing, then the airway might be obstructed and should be repositioned. A jaw-thrust can help to lift the tongue away from the posterior airway. A nasopharyngeal airway can be inserted to aid in oxygenation and respiration. If they remain apneic, BVM assistance may be needed. A pulse should be checked at the onset of the seizure, as fatal arrhythmias may cause clonic activity due to cerebral anoxia and would require the initiation of CPR.[4]

In some situations, the patient may not need to be transported to the hospital. If the athlete has known epilepsy, the seizure lasts less than 5 minutes, and they recover relatively quickly and then emergency department (ED) evaluation may not be necessary. However, if the athlete is recovering slowly, has a second seizure, a seizure lasting greater than 5 minutes, or does not have diagnosed seizure disorder, then emergency department evaluation is appropriate.[3] Family members may be helpful in characterizing whether a seizure and recovery period is typical for the athlete, as well as administering rescue medications if they have the prescription for the patient available. Once emergency medical services (EMS) arrives, they may administer abortive medications such as midazolam, diazepam, or lorazepam.

Once the seizure stops, the patient may be somnolent in the minutes immediately following and may require temporary respiratory support including jaw-thrust or even NPA placement. They should gradually become more alert and return to their baseline. A failure to return to baseline or a second seizure would necessitate EMS transport to the emergency department.

High Cervical Spine Injury

Cervical spine injury can lead to airway compromise due to impaired intercostal muscle strength, impaired abdominal muscle strength, and in injuries above C5, diaphragm paralysis. In the period immediately following spinal cord injury, spinal shock can develop and complete loss of function below the injury can occur, leading to rapid airway compromise in high cervical injury.[5] The diaphragm is innervated by cervical spinal levels C3-5, so injury to or above these levels can lead to diaphragm weakness, paralysis, lower tidal volumes, and ineffective ventilation. Rarely, complete apnea can occur. In cervical injuries below C5, respiration can still be compromised due to intercostal and abdominal muscle weakness.[6] These athletes may demonstrate increased work of breathing, tachypnea, and ineffective chest rise.[5]

All of those with suspected cervical spine injury should have their cervical spine stabilized throughout the assessment, airway intervention, and transport. Obtunded athletes may appear apneic due to obstructed airway, and this apnea will improve with airway maneuvers or airway adjunct usage. Athletes with suspected cervical injury who do not improve with airway repositioning may require BVM respirations. If the athlete is breathing but with increased work of breathing or very little chest rise, breaths can be assisted with BVM by giving a breath when the athlete initiates spontaneous respiration. This provides respiratory support by giving positive pressure which increases lung tidal volume and ventilation. In completely apneic athletes, one breath should be given every 6 seconds. Ventilation with BVM can be improved by insertion of oral pharyngeal airway, nasopharyngeal airway, or supraglottic airway until EMS transport arrives.

Upper Airway

Anaphylaxis

Symptoms of anaphylaxis include rash or hives, shortness of breath and wheezing, abdominal pain, vomiting, and swelling of the face, oropharynx, and lower airway, as well as hypotension. Classification of an allergic reaction as anaphylaxis requires symptoms in two different body systems: skin, pulmonary, cardiovascular, and gastrointestinal (GI). Symptoms do not progress in a predictable pattern; an athlete can progress rapidly from mild rash to airway swelling and hypotension.

As soon as anaphylaxis is suspected, EMS should be called and a dose of intramuscular (IM) epinephrine of 0.01 mg/kg of 1:1000 epinephrine (1 mg/mL) should be given. Maximum dose for adults is 0.5 mg and 0.3 mg for children.[7] This is ideally administered using an epinephrine auto-injector (such as Epi Pen), however appropriately dosed epinephrine in pre-drawn syringes is also suitable. The pen should be held against the athlete's thigh or another large muscle group. The plunger can then be depressed and the pen held to the skin for 3 seconds. Take care to ensure that the needle is pointed toward the athlete rather than the physician's thumb, as accidental injection of the administrator has been reported.

Absorption has been proven fastest when administered in the lateral thigh, however, if the athlete is in the extremis and equipment blocking the thigh would take significant time to remove, the initial dose can be given in another large muscle group such as the upper arm.[8] Failure to hold to the skin will result in too small of a dose administered. If there is no or little improvement in symptoms, a second dose of epinephrine can be administered 5 minutes after the first. Every athlete who is given a dose of epinephrine should be transported to the emergency department for cardiac monitoring and observation to ensure that symptoms do not rebound.

Because of the rapid progression of symptoms in anaphylaxis, early administration of epinephrine is key. Therefore, it is important to know the medical history of the team, and have an Epi Pen available if any have a known history of allergic reaction or anaphylaxis. In the absence of any known allergies, epinephrine remains an important component of the sideline medical bag. Other adjuncts in addition to epinephrine administration include albuterol for wheezing, diphenhydramine (eg, Benadryl), and famotidine (eg, Pepcid) for their anti-histamine properties. Antihistamines improve cutaneous symptoms, but do not do anything to reverse the cardiovascular or pulmonary symptoms of anaphylaxis, and their utility has been questioned.[7] Steroids may be given upon arrival in the emergency department, although there is also conflicting evidence of their utility.[9]

In the worst case, the airway swelling associated with anaphylaxis can be catastrophic leading to eventual respiratory arrest from airway obstruction. Swelling of the lips, tongue, uvula, and other posterior oropharynx structures can occur, as well as swelling of the hypopharynx and epiglottis. This swelling can make oxygenation incredibly difficult and airway adjuncts such as oral airways, nasal airways, and supraglottic devices difficult to place and at times ineffective. For this reason, early epinephrine administration and prompt transport to an emergency department are critical.

Exam of an athlete with suspected anaphylaxis should include a thorough skin exam to look for evidence of rash and hives, lung auscultation for wheezing or stridor, and observation for any signs of respiratory distress such as increased respiratory rate, intercostal or subcostal retractions, or pursed lip breathing. The abdomen should be palpated for tenderness. The oropharynx should be examined for any sign of edema in the lips, tongue, or uvula. The athlete should be asked to speak to see if they have any evidence of hoarseness indicating swelling of the vocal cords and hypopharynx. Symptoms or exam findings in two systems or any evidence of airway swelling, respiratory distress, or circulatory collapse should prompt epinephrine administration and EMS call for transport. If the athlete has an isolated rash, diphenhydramine can be administered and close monitoring for progression is appropriate.

Foreign body

There are little to no data on foreign body aspiration in sports, and events are likely uncommon. Foreign body aspiration should be suspected when an athlete has sudden onset choking, stridor, and dyspnea, especially if the athlete was just engaged in an activity that could have caused aspiration, such as eating, or facial trauma that may have caused tooth fracture and aspiration.

Larger foreign bodies often lodge in the oropharynx or hypopharynx above the vocal cords. If these larger objects are completely obstructive, the athlete will be unable to phonate. Smaller foreign bodies can be aspirated into the bronchi, and in that case, unilateral wheezing or decreased breath sounds may be heard. In children, even small objects can have a profound effect on breathing due to the small caliber of their airways.[10] Foreign body aspiration, especially of larger objects, can lead to quick progression of loss of consciousness and death if the obstruction is not relieved swiftly. Aspiration into the lower airways can cause airway spasm and edema, so dyspnea and hypoxia may worsen with time.

The sideline physician should evaluate the airway, first by looking in the oropharynx to check for any visible foreign body. Visible foreign body should be removed, but blind finger sweeps should be avoided as they can push objects farther into the airway. The athlete should be evaluated for any evidence of stridor, wheezing, and decreased breath sounds. Observe for evidence of increased work of breathing, such as intercostal and subcostal retractions and tracheal tugging.

Athletes who can still phonate should be allowed to try and clear their own airway by coughing. If the athlete cannot clear phonate or cough, then steps must be taken by the provider to try to clear the obstruction. For choking children and adults, abdominal thrusts should be performed (aka the Heimlich maneuver) until the airway clears and the athlete can breathe again, or they lose consciousness. If they lose consciousness, they should be laid supine, ideally on a hard service, and chest compressions should be started according to Basic Life Support. Every 15 to 30 compressions, the airway should be checked for a foreign object, and the object should be removed if visualized. Again, avoid blind finger sweeps as this may result in the object being pushed farther into the airway.

If the sideline physician is comfortable and the proper equipment is available, direct laryngoscopy can be attempted, and if the foreign body is visualized, an attempt at removal can be made. Magill forceps are ideal for grasping foreign bodies in the hypopharynx under direct visualization. Objects or substances that have been aspirated into the lower airway cannot be removed and will likely require bronchoscopy at the hospital. If the provider cannot remove the object and is confident that it is supraglottic, then a cricothyrotomy can be performed to bypass the obstructed upper airway, or jet ventilation through a needle cricothyrotomy in children less than 12 years old.

Facial trauma

Significant facial trauma can cause emergent airway issues, especially in the case of significant bleeding or substantial mandibular fracture. Incidence of facial fracture in sport has been cited as anywhere between 4% and 20% and most common mechanism depends on the popularity of various sports within an area.[11] Football, hockey, soccer, and baseball are the most common sports implicated in facial fracture in the United States.[12] Collisions with other players or other sporting equipment (such as a ball or puck) are the most common cause of facial fractures. Fractures of the lower and middle thirds of the face are most common, as these are often left unprotected by sporting equipment.[12] Incidence of significant bleeding or airway obstruction in facial trauma has been cited to be anywhere between 2% and 6% of all patients with maxillofacial trauma, however, studies have included all mechanisms of facial trauma, and there are a paucity of data surrounding necessity of airway management in sport-related facial fracture.[13]

Facial fractures can be complicated by their association with head and neck injury. In-line cervical stabilization should be maintained whenever possible if the athlete is having midline neck pain or is unconscious. However, if the athlete is awake and the cervical spine can be cleared, a seated position or other position of comfort can often avoid many of the airway complications associated with facial trauma—namely aspiration of blood and obstruction of the oropharynx by the tongue.

The tongue is attached to the anterior mandible and anterior mandibular fractures can cause the tongue to shift posteriorly causing an upper airway obstruction.[14] A jaw-thrust can often relieve this obstruction by shifting the tongue more anteriorly again, however, with bilateral mandibular fractures, this may be ineffective due to disruption of the communication between the anterior mandible and the angle. If jaw-thrust is ineffective and does not appear to move the anterior mandible, manual anterior traction of the jaw and tongue should be attempted. If the athlete is unconscious, an oral airway can be attempted. Nasal airways should be avoided if significant mid-face trauma is suspected as there is theoretic risk of entrance into the calvarium through a mid-face fracture. Maxillary fractures (also known as LeFort fractures) are much less common, however can be associated with increased risk of severe bleeding, and posterior displacement can also cause upper airway obstruction.[12]

There can be significant associated bleeding due to mucosal disruption, however, most will improve with direct pressure achieved by biting on gauze. Rarely, bleeding will be so severe that interventional radiology (IR) embolization is required.[15] Mandibular fractures can also cause sublingual hematoma, soft tissue swelling, significant dental disruption, and bleeding, all of which can lead to oropharyngeal obstruction requiring definitive airway management. These sequelae can make orotracheal intubation difficult due to difficulty with visualization of the airway, and may necessitate surgical airway placement.

Lower Airway

Asthma

Rates of asthma have been consistently shown to be higher among athletes than the general population. Team physicians should be aware if any athletes have a history of asthma and have the appropriate equipment to assess and treat them immediately. Each athlete should have an albuterol inhaler for use, ideally with a spacer. A peak flow meter is also helpful for guiding decision making on treatment and return to play.

Up to 50% to 90% of athletes with history of asthma experience some degree of bronchoconstriction during exercise.[16] Adequate chronic control of an athlete's asthma is the most important factor in preventing the need for sideline intervention, however, even with good control, asthma exacerbations can occur. Ideally peak expiratory flow (PEF) measures should be obtained during athlete's pre-participation to be used as a baseline for comparison in times of exacerbation.

Athletes exhibiting signs of bronchoconstriction or airway hyper-reactivity such as increased work of breathing, chest tightness, cough, and wheezing, should be removed from play and PEF should be measured. If PEF is decreased by 10% to 15% from baseline, then they should be given two puffs of their short-acting beta-2 agonist inhaler, most commonly albuterol. Inhalers are best administered with spacers to allow adequate aerosolization of the medication and delivery to the lower airway. Symptoms typically improve within 5 minutes of inhaler use and PEF should be re-measured at that time. If symptoms have not improved and the PEF is not back to baseline, another two puffs can be given.[17]

The athlete can return to competition after PEF returns to baseline and they are feeling symptomatically improved. If symptoms do not improve after a total of four puffs of albuterol, or if symptoms worsen at any point, transport should be initiated to a higher level of care. Depending on the degree of respiratory distress that the patient is experiencing, this could mean transport to the nearest emergency department or back to the athletic training room. If athletes are exhibiting signs of significant respiratory distress such as intercostal/subcostal retractions, significant tachypnea, the inability to speak in full sentences, or sitting in a "tripoding" position and this does not improve significantly with albuterol administration, EMS should be called and transport should be initiated to the local emergency department.

Laryngotracheal injury

Trauma to the throat and larynx is less common than facial trauma in sport, however, injuries can be difficult to diagnose and at times life-threatening.[8] The neck is left relatively vulnerable to injury in most sports and can be struck in collisions with other players or playing equipment.

The larynx has three main purposes: breathing, phonation, and airway protection during swallowing. The cricoid cartilage is found at the inferior-most portion of the larynx. It forms a full ring around the airway and supports the arytenoid cartilages and small muscles that move the vocal cords allowing for phonation.[18] The thyroid cartilage, or "Adams apple," protects the larynx anteriorly. The epiglottis lies above the vocal cords and covers them during swallowing to protect from aspiration. The hyoid bone is the superior-most structure of the larynx.[18] Any of these structures can be injured with blunt trauma, with even small injuries causing significant alterations in function of the larynx.

Blunt trauma or penetrating trauma to the laryngeal structures can result in swelling, hematoma, cartilage or bony fracture, mucosal injury, recurrent laryngeal nerve injury, or even complete laryngotracheal separation.

Sideline evaluation should always include a cervical exam due to the association between laryngeal and cervical injury. The airway should be assessed for any signs of impending airway collapse such as increased work of breathing, tachypnea, and significant stridor.[19] If the athlete is in significant respiratory distress, emergency transfer for definitive management is advised as the usual methods for securing an airway in the field can cause worsening trauma. Supraglottic airways carry risk of further disrupting an injured larynx as does direct laryngoscopy.

In an athlete requiring ventilation on the sideline, attempts should be made using bag-valve mask and oral or nasal airway if necessary, ideally avoiding the insertion of supraglottic airway or endotracheal (ET) tube if possible unless absolutely necessary. Cricothyrotomy also carries significant risk and may be more difficult than anticipated due to altered anatomy from the injury.[18] Surgical tracheostomy is generally considered the safest option for airway management with significant laryngeal injury, however, this is unlikely to be feasible on the sideline due to provider comfort and equipment available.[20] If available, video laryngoscopy, such as portable GlideScope, may be safer than direct laryngoscopy.[19] However, for those who do not routinely perform intubation, it may be difficult to distinguish normal from abnormal appearance of the laryngeal structures, making it difficult to determine if intubation is safe.

Concerning symptoms after laryngeal trauma include hoarseness, dysphonia/ aphonia, dysphagia, odynophagia, cough, stridor, dyspnea, and respiratory distress. Hemoptysis and hematemesis can also occur. The athlete should be observed for respiratory distress, drooling, loss of normal laryngeal architecture (loss of prominence of Adam's apple), lacerations, and any ecchymosis in the area. The neck should be palpated for subcutaneous emphysema, tenderness, and tracheal placement at the midline. Any bubbling of blood or air movement through a laceration is concerning for laryngotracheal injury, as is subcutaneous emphysema.[18]

Any of the above symptoms or physical exam findings should prompt transfer for higher level of care and evaluation in an emergency department. Workup will often include computed tomography (CT) scan of the neck and fiberoptic laryngoscopy for direct visualization of the larynx.[20] Common findings on laryngoscopy include vocal cord hematoma, edema, hematoma of surrounding soft tissues, vocal cord paralysis, or avulsion.[19]

Many patients will undergo 24-hour observation for worsening airway compromise. Conservative therapy usually includes humidified air and elevation of the head of the bed.[18] Steroids and anti-reflux medication may also be given.[19]

SUMMARY

Emergent airway issues in sports are rare occurrences. However, when airway compromise happens, the sideline physician will be relied upon to rapidly assess and manage the airway. There are many conditions that can lead to airway compromise, including significant head or facial trauma, medical emergencies such as seizure, hypoglycemia, or cardiac arrest, and pulmonary and laryngotracheal trauma, but general assessment and management principles are the same. An athlete who is awake and speaking has at least a momentarily patent airway. The downed and unconscious athlete should be presumed to have airway obstruction and a head-tilt chin-lift maneuver or jaw-thrust should be attempted. If this does not relieve obstruction, then an airway adjunct such as an NPA, OPA, or supraglottic airway can be inserted if no significant pharyngeal trauma is suspected. The apneic athlete will require BVM ventilation with the possible addition of other airway adjuncts. In very rare cases, intubation or surgical airway may be required if the sideline physician is comfortable with the practice.

CLINICS CARE POINTS

- The initial approach to airway management and intervention focuses on the assessment of three basic considerations: failure to oxygenate, failure to ventilate, and failure to maintain airway patency.

- The differential diagnosis for airway emergency can be divided into several classes to aid in identifying the etiology of respiratory distress or airway compromise: obtundation/apnea, upper airway compromise, and lower airway compromise.

- A simple airway positioning maneuver is often sufficient to establish airway patency in an unconscious athlete. The two most common methods for opening the airway are the head-tilt/chin-lift and jaw-thrust maneuvers.

- Various airway adjuncts can be used if airway repositioning fails including an OPA, NPA, and supraglottic devices. If these fail, intubation or surgical airway may be necessary.

- The sideline physician should know the medical history of their athletes to be better prepared for possible sideline airway emergencies including the history of seizures, allergies, and asthma. They should also have appropriate medications such as albuterol and epinephrine available to deal with airway emergencies caused by medical conditions such as asthma and anaphylaxis.

DISCLOSURE

The authors have nothing to disclose.

REFERENCES

1. Bielski A, Rivas E, Ruetzler K, et al. Comparison of blind intubation via supraglottic airway devices versus standard intubation during different airway emergency scenarios in inexperienced hand: Randomized, crossover manikin trial. Medicine (Baltim) 2018;97(40):e12593.
2. Capovilla G, Kaufman KR, Perucca E, et al. Epilepsy, seizures, physical exercise, and sports: A report from the IL AE Task Force on Sports and Epilepsy. Epilepsia 2016;57(1):6–12.
3. O'Hara KA. First aid for seizures: the impotance of education and appropriate response. J Child Neurol 2007;22(5):30S–7S.
4. Sabu J, Regeti K, Mallappallil M, et al. Convulsive Syncope Induced by Ventricular Arrhythmia Masquerading as Epileptic Seizures: Case Report and Literature Review. J Clin Med Res 2016;8(8):610–5.
5. Berlowitz DJ, Wadsworth B, Ross J. Respiratory problems and management in people with spinal cord injury. Breathe 2016;12(4):328–40.
6. Schilero GJ, Bauman WA, Radulovic M. Traumatic Spinal Cord Injury: Pulmonary Physiologic Principles and Management. Clin Chest Med 2018;39(2):411–25.
7. Zilberstein J, McCurdy MT, Winters ME. Anaphylaxis. J Emerg Med 2014;47(2): 182–7.
8. Simons FE, Gu X, Simons KJ. Epinephrine absorption in adults: intramuscular versus subcutaneous injection. J Allergy Clin Immunol 2001;108(5):871–3.

9. Choo KJ, Simons E, Sheikh A. Glucocorticoids for the treatment of anaphylaxis: Cochrane systematic review. Allergy 2010;65(10):1205–11.
10. Brady MF, Burns B. Airway obstruction. Treasure Island (FL): StatPearls Publishing; 2022.
11. Puolakkainen T, Murros OJ, Abio A, et al. Sports-based distribution of facial fractures - findings from a four-season country. Acta Odontol Scand 2022;80(3): 191–6.
12. Viozzi CF. Maxillofacial and Mandibular Fractures in Sports. Clin Sports Med 2017;36(2):355–68.
13. Tung T-C, Tseng W-S, Lai J-P, et al. Acute Life-Threatening Injuries in Facial Fracture Patients: A Review of 1025 Patients. J Trauma 2000;49:420–4.
14. Lainhart J, Toldi J, Tennison M. Facial Trauma in Sports. Curr Sports Med Rep 2017;16(1):23–9.
15. Dar P, Gupta P, Kaul RP, et al. Haemorrhage control beyond Advanced Trauma Life Support (ATLS) protocol in life threatening maxillofacial trauma - experience from a level trauma centre. Br J Oral Maxillofac Surg 2021;59(6):700–4.
16. Olympia RP, Brady J. Emergency preparedness in high school-based athletics: a review of the literature and recommendations for sport health professionals. Phys Sportsmed 2013;41(2):15–25.
17. Allen TW. Sideline Management of Asthma. Curr Sports Med Rep 2005;4:301–4.
18. SA P, CD L. Laryngeal Trauma in Sport. Curr Sports Med Rep 2008;7(1):16–21.
19. Mendis D, Anderson JA. Blunt laryngeal trauma secondary to sporting injuries. J Laryngol Otol 2017;131(8):728–35.
20. Schaefer SD. Management of acute blunt and penetrating external laryngeal trauma. Laryngoscope 2014;124(1):233–44.

Chest and Thorax Injuries in Athletes

Alexander J. Tomesch, MD, CAQ-SM[a],*, Matthew Negaard, MD, CAQ-SM[b,c], Olivia Keller-Baruch, MD[a]

KEYWORDS

- Pneumothorax • Pneumomediastinum • Rib fracture • Thoracic vascular injury
- Blunt cardiac injury • Sternoclavicular joint dislocation

KEY POINTS

- Chest injuries are infrequent, but can be life-threatening when they occur.
- There are physical exam will lend clues to help diagnose many different emergent thoracic injuries in athletes.
- Ultrasound is a useful tool to help differentiate thoracic injuries from blunt trauma.

PNEUMOTHORAX

Introduction

Traumatic pneumothorax (PTX) is an injury sustained after blunt trauma often caused by a displaced rib fracture puncturing the visceral pleura.[1] PTX in sports is rare with incidence limited to case series and case reports, however, has been described in multiple sports including football, rugby, soccer, ice hockey, weightlifting, and scuba.[2,3] PTX can be a life-threatening injury, thus, must be quickly diagnosed and treated.

Patient Evaluation Overview

Athletes with trauma to the chest endorsing pleuritic chest pain and dyspnea should be evaluated for the presence of PTX.[4] On physical exam, there is often decreased breath sounds on the side of the PTX, however, this may be difficult to assess on the sideline. Therefore, athletes with suspected PTX should be evaluated in a quiet space.[2,4] Unstable vital signs, hypoxia, distended neck veins, or tracheal deviation may all be indicative of a tension pneumothorax and should be emergently transported to the nearest emergency department (ED).[2,4]

[a] Department of Emergency Medicine, University of Missouri, Columbia, MO, USA; [b] Department of Emergency Medicine, University of Iowa, Iowa City, IA, USA; [c] Forte Sports Medicine and Orthopedics, Indianapolis, IN, USA
* Corresponding author. University of Missouri, 1 Hospital Drive, Columbia, MO 65201.
E-mail address: alex.tomesch@gmail.com
Twitter: @DocTomesch (A.J.T.); @MattNegaard (M.N.)

Clin Sports Med 42 (2023) 385–400
https://doi.org/10.1016/j.csm.2023.03.001
0278-5919/23/Published by Elsevier Inc.
sportsmed.theclinics.com

PTX can be diagnosed with chest x-ray (CXR) as well as ultrasound (US). US has been shown to have a higher sensitivity (ranging from 86% to 98%) when compared to a supine CXR (sensitivities ranging from 28% to 75%).[5] Given the portability and test characteristics, US is the preferred modality to diagnose PTX in the sideline setting.

Medical Treatment Options

If PTX is suspected or confirmed on the sideline, supplemental oxygen should be administered immediately.[2] Definitive treatment of a PTX often depends on the size of the PTX. PTX making up less than 15% of the total lung volume often requires no treatment and can be observed.[1] For injuries that make up greater than 20% of total lung volume, a chest tube or catheter will likely be required for evacuation.[1]

If the athlete is showing signs and symptoms of a tension pneumothorax or shows unstable vital signs, an emergent needle decompression should be performed to convert the tension PTX into a simple PTX.[2] Traditionally, needle decompression is performed by inserting a 5 cm large bore angio catheter (14 gauge or larger) in the second intercostal space in the mid-clavicular line, just above the superior edge of the rib. Needle decompression success relies on the ability to reach the pleural space, and larger individuals may have a chest wall thickness which exceeds the catheter length. An alternative site of needle decompression is the fourth to fifth intercostal space in the anterior to mid-axillary line as the chest wall is thinner at this location.[6]

New Developments

Point of care US is becoming increasingly more common for the evaluation of blunt chest trauma including diagnosis of PTX.[4,5]

Evaluation of Outcome and/or Long-Term Recommendations

There are no guidelines on return to sport recommendations after a traumatic PTX. However, most experts agree that there should be a resolution of the PTX radiographically before any exertional athletic activities can resume.[1,2] It is also suggested that athletes undergo a supervised gradual return to sport progression with most athletes being able to return to sports 4 weeks after resolution of the PTX.[1]

A PTX is a contraindication for air travel and most guidelines recommend a delay of up to 14 days post-resolution of the PTX before air travel.[7]

SUMMARY/DISCUSSION/FUTURE DIRECTIONS

Traumatic PTX is a serious complication of blunt trauma that is rare but can occur in various sports. It can have potentially life-threatening implications, and thus must be quickly diagnosed and properly managed. The use of US to diagnose a traumatic PTX is the most sensitive tool to use on the sideline or in a remote setting. There are currently no guidelines on the return to play after a PTX which could be a target for future research.

CLINICS CARE POINTS

- US is a sensitive and portable tool to accurately diagnose a pneumothorax.
- Supplemental oxygen should be applied to anyone with suspected or confirmed pneumothorax.
- Definitive treatment of a pneumothorax will be determined by the size of the injury.
- If a tension pneumothorax is clinically suspected, needle decompression should be performed.
- Air travel should be delayed after sustaining a pneumothorax.

PNEUMOMEDIASTINUM
Introduction

Pneumomediastinum (PM), the presence of air within the mediastinum, is a rare condition that can also occur in athletes. These injuries can occur either via direct trauma, or spontaneously. Spontaneous PM has a reported incidence rate of 0.001% to 0.01% of all adult inpatients.[8] In children with asthma visiting the ED, there is an incidence of 0.3%.[8] PM has been reported in scuba diving, weightlifting, running, soccer, football, ice hockey, and snorkeling.[2] It has been proposed that traumatic PM in collision sports may occur due to Valsalva forces during collision rather than direct injury to the trachea or bronchus.[9] These injuries typically heal well with conservative treatment, but still warrant close monitoring and require a high level of suspicion to diagnose.

Patient Evaluation Overview

Unfortunately for PM, there is no tell-tale symptom or physical exam finding that will clue the provider into this diagnosis. Most patients will complain of some sort of chest discomfort. The most common findings included subcutaneous emphysema (crepitus), substernal pain, dyspnea, odynophagia, and cough.[9] The most specific sign is Hamman crunch, or crunching murmur heard with each heartbeat, indicative of free air in the mediastinum.[9] This was still only present in 12% to 56% of people with PM depending on the study evaluated.[9] Once there is a high index of suspicion for this diagnosis, imaging must be obtained.

Simple CXR is the first study of choice. CXR helps rule out other potential causes of chest pain in the athlete (chest wall fracture, pneumothorax, pulmonary contusion) and can provide additional diagnoses as well. In one small case series, diagnosis was made on 12 of 13 CXR.[10] Findings used for diagnosis on CXR include air streaks in the superior mediastinum, prominent heart silhouette, and subcutaneous emphysema.[8] However, to determine the cause or location of the leak, computed tomography (CT) should be obtained.

Additionally, an electrocardiogram (EKG) can have findings associated with PM. The most common findings are the loss of R wave in precordial leads, decrease in voltages, and ST elevation in inferior leads.[11–17] This is postulated to be caused by stretching of the myocardium which leads to narrowing of the coronary arteries (ST elevation) or stretching of the pericardium which can present a pericarditis-type picture on EKG.[11]

Pharmacologic or Medical Treatment Options

Typically, once patients have PM diagnosed, subspecialists may recommend additional testing to further evaluate for the cause or source of the PM such as bronchoscopy, or esophagram. Often, observation is the primary treatment of this injury. Pain control is important. Oxygen therapy has been suggested for nitrogen washout as in pneumothorax, however, there are no definitive data that this is helpful for PM.[8] Antibiotics and dietary changes are additional interventions that are typically employed, however, there again are no definitive data that they improve outcomes.[2,8,9]

Non-Pharmacologic or Surgical/Interventional Treatment Options

As described above, treatment is typically with observation and supportive care. However, if there is concern for significant traumatic tracheobronchial injury with respiratory compromise, aggressive care may be indicated with intubation. Thankfully, this is almost never the case in PM with blunt trauma (0.1%).[2]

Combination Therapies

None.

Treatment Resistance/Complications

If a patient's symptoms are relatively well controlled after diagnosis and there are no additional concerning signs on exam or imaging, patients may be able to be monitored outside of the hospital with close follow-up. However, if there are any concerns, a short admission for observation is reasonable.

Evaluation of Outcome and/or Long-Term Recommendations

For athletes with PM who are discharged from the hospital, careful consideration is used to determine when it is safe to fly again. Following pneumothorax, it is recommended to delay travel for at least 14 days after resolution. There are no such guidelines for PM. A survey of thoracic surgeons resulted in about half recommending a waiting period of 14 days after resolution, and the other half were agreeable to flight with some remnant of PM.[2]

Returning to sports following PM has limited data. Most opinions available suggest a relatively quick return after resolution of symptoms, including to contact sports.

SUMMARY/DISCUSSION/FUTURE DIRECTIONS

PM is an overall very rare condition, but can happen in a wide variety of athletes. Most PM that occurs even within the scope of collision sports is likely spontaneous in nature. Careful evaluation of these patients with imaging is needed to determine the extent of the injury with concomitant observation inpatient versus close outpatient follow-up if symptoms are controllable. Patients should be able to return to sports and air travel relatively quickly after PM, though there are limited data on this. Follow-up study on return to sports and air travel would be an interesting and valuable study in the future.

CLINICS CARE POINTS

- PM is a rare diagnosis and even less common in athletics
- Even if occurring in a collision sport, the cause is likely secondary to a spontaneous PM
- Common symptoms include subcutaneous emphysema, substernal chest pain, dyspnea, odynophagia, and cough
- Hamman sign is most specific, however, only occurs 12% to 5% of the time
- EKG changes can occur secondary to PM
- Treatment is primarily supportive care
  - Oxygen, antibiotics, and dietary changes have been suggested, but there are limited to no data to support this
- Return to sports and air travel is again limited to expert opinion, but athletes can likely start back into activities following the resolution of symptoms

RIB FRACTURES
Introduction

Acute rib fractures occur with significant blunt trauma to the thorax. To our knowledge, there is no published incidence of acute rib fractures in sports, however, there is extensive literature on stress fractures of the ribs in various sports.[18] Rib fractures often result in significant pain limiting athletic performance. There are also significant, potentially life-threatening complications associated with rib fractures such as pneumothorax, pulmonary conditions, and pneumonia.

Patient Evaluation Overview

Athletes with trauma to the chest with isolated pain over one or more ribs should have a high suspicion of a rib fracture. CXR has often been used to diagnose rib fractures, however, has been shown to have very poor sensitivity, as low as 24% in one study.[19] CXR may be useful to help evaluate for complications of rib fractures such as pulmonary contusions and pneumothorax. However, US has been shown to have a higher sensitivity (80%) in detecting rib fractures. It is also useful in diagnosing the aforementioned complications of rib fractures.[19] The transportability and ability to use US on the sidelines make it the preferred method to diagnose acute rib fractures in the athlete. US test characteristics will be dependent on the skillset of the operator and increase with proficiency and experience.

Pharmacologic or Medical Treatment Options

Adequate pain control in rib fractures is not only important to allow the athlete to return to sport, but also decrease the risk of pneumonia after sustaining a rib fracture.[20] Pain control is generally attempted with oral and topical nonsteroidal anti-inflammatory drugs (NSAIDs). Opioids can also be used for pain control, but will limit athletic participation. Topical lidocaine in the form of patches and creams has been shown to be useful in conjunction with other non-opioid medications to assist in pain control of rib fractures.[21] Rib blocks, the use of anesthetic medications injected at the site of the rib fracture, are often used in sports for pain control. In the ED setting, several different plane blocks including the serratus anterior plane block and erector spinae plane block have been described to achieve analgesia from rib fractures.[22,23]

Non-Pharmacologic Treatment Options

Kinesio Taping in conjunction with NSAIDs has been shown to improve pain in patients with isolated rib fractures in the ED setting.[24] Rib belts have also been shown to improve pain, however, some have cautioned their uses as they may limit respiratory function.[25]

Treatment Resistance/Complications

Acute complications of rib fractures include pneumothorax, hemothorax, and pulmonary contusions.[26] The most common delayed complication from rib fractures is pneumonia.[27]

New Developments

Point-of-care US is now more frequently used to diagnose rib fractures as well as the complications associated with rib fractures, such as pneumothorax. Additionally, US can be used in the treatment of rib fractures through isolated rib and chest wall plane blocks.[22,23]

Evaluation of Outcome and/or Long-Term Recommendations

There are no guidelines or consensus recommendations on return to sport for athletes who have sustained one or more rib fractures. However, if there are no other associated injuries and pain is adequately controlled, athletes can often return to sport quickly with a protective device.

SUMMARY/DISCUSSION/FUTURE DIRECTIONS

There is a paucity of literature on the epidemiology, diagnosis, and management of acute, traumatic rib fractures in athletes. However, we can extrapolate from the Emergency Medicine and Trauma literature the diagnosis and management of traumatic rib fractures. Future investigation into the management of these injuries in athletes of different sports may lead to different approaches to best treat rib fractures in different types of athletes.

CLINICS CARE POINTS

- US is a sensitive and portable modality to diagnose rib fractures and associated complications.
- The addition of kinesio tape to NSAIDs may provide increased pain relief in treating rib fractures.
- US-guided injections can assist in pain control for rib fractures.
- Adequate pain control decreases the long-term complications of rib fractures.

VASCULAR INJURY
Introduction

Blunt thoracic vascular injury is a rare event in any patient, most commonly caused by high-velocity mechanisms such as motor vehicle collisions. These injuries can occur in athletes as well. They have been described in skiing, rugby, weightlifting, football, and paragliding accidents.[28–33] Injuries most commonly occur as dissection of the aorta, however, superior vena cava tear, aortic rupture, and coronary artery dissection have also been described. Although these injuries are not common, they are life-threatening and require a high level of suspicion to diagnose. Historically, these are very deadly injuries with only about 15% of patients making it out of the pre-hospital setting.[32]

Patient Evaluation Overview

Providers should have the highest concern for thoracic vascular injury in patients who sustain high-velocity collisions such as in downhill skiing, football, race car driving, or paragliding. When approaching the patient, remember to follow the ABCs. This is essentially a trauma patient and deserves a thorough primary and secondary survey. In the case of thoracic vascular injury, the first clue may be related to a pulse deficit. First, consider if there is a difference in intensity of contralateral radial pulses, but also consider if there is a significant pulse deficit from the radial pulse to the dorsalis pedis or posterior tibial pulse (referred to as pseudo coarctation syndrome). This often will be logistically more difficult in some athletes, but important to consider if still unsure of injury diagnosis immediately. Pseudo coarctation syndrome can be present in up to 53% of patients in the acute setting with palpation of pulses, and 56% of patients when taking blood pressure measurements.[32]

The most common symptoms of patients with thoracic aortic rupture include dyspnea, back pain, dysphagia, and cough.[34] Other signs on physical exam include chest wall contusion, pulse changes (as outlined above), and systolic murmur at the base of the heart or between the scapula.[34] However, up to 30% of patients may have no symptoms or signs of injury to the chest.[34] If pulse deficit or high level of concern for a thoracic vascular injury is found, the patient needs to be immediately transported to the nearest hospital, preferably with vascular or cardiothoracic surgery.

Once at the hospital, patients need to undergo CT angiography. This is the gold standard of diagnosis of aortic injury, and is recommended by the Eastern Association of Trauma (EAST) trauma guidelines as first-line imaging.[35] In one meta-analysis, 92.7% of patients with thoracic aortic rupture from blunt trauma had an abnormality of the mediastinum on CXR.[36,37] CXR can be performed, and if it does not show any abnormalities, it significantly lowers the likelihood of injury,[34] however, it is not completely sensitive, and this is why CT is mandated.

Medical Treatment Options

At this time, there is no medication that can fix a vascular injury; however, some medications prevent the worsening of a dissection or extravasation. The patient's blood pressure should be managed to a normotensive to slightly hypotensive level.[28,32] Systolic blood pressure of 90 mm Hg is appropriate. Patients should not be given fluid or blood products in the field if their blood pressure is holding above this. Additionally, if they are hypertensive or high normotensive, they should be considered for induction of hypotension with short-acting medications like esmolol. Heart rate control is preferred and therefore esmolol should be first line over other blood pressure-lowering agents (nitroglycerine, hydralazine) which may induce reflex tachycardia.

Surgical intervention is the final stage of treatment of aortic dissection.

New Developments

If US is available, performing a rapid US for shock and hypotension exam on the patient can help narrow the differential diagnosis. This does evaluate for intra-abdominal causes as well but does focus on several causes for hypotension within the chest. The exam includes imaging of the

1. Heart (Parasternal long, apical four chamber)
2. Inferior vena cava (IVC)
3. Morrison's pouch with hemothorax view
4. Splenorenal recess with hemothorax view
5. Bladder
6. Aorta
7. Bilateral pulmonary view

This exam is essentially an Extended Focused Assessment with Sonography in Trauma (E-FAST) with views of the Inferior Vena Cava (IVC), more focused views of the heart, and aorta. Unfortunately, the thoracic aorta is difficult to assess with bedside US and is a limiting factor, however, one can potentially visualize intrathoracic injury with a dissection flap into the heart, or the abdominal aorta. This exam will take time to perfect, but in an experienced operator's hands, this can provide a lot of information in a short period to help with identifying the injury.

Evaluation of Outcome and/or Long-Term Recommendations

Up to 85% of people who suffer blunt traumatic thoracic vascular injury do not survive transport to a hospital. If the patient is fortunate enough to make it to the hospital, they will have to undergo surgical repair. They will have a long recovery to get back to a functional baseline. It is unlikely that an athlete who has suffered a major vascular injury will return to play, however, not impossible and will have to be considered on a case-by-case basis. There has been a football player who with a vena cava tear that was able to return to play.

SUMMARY/DISCUSSION/FUTURE DIRECTIONS

Traumatic thoracic vascular injury is a rare, but often life-threatening injury. Oftentimes patients with these types of injuries do not make it to the hospital setting due to the severity of this disease process. Pulse pressure deficits are the most likely indication on the sideline of potential vascular injury. In the pre-hospital setting, it is important to maintain normal blood pressure to even hypotension if the thoracic vascular injury is considered. Point of care ultrasound (POCUS) can be quite helpful in aiding in the diagnosis of injuries if available and the operator has experience. Once patients arrive at the hospital, definitive imaging with CT angiogram, and then subsequent surgery, is indicated for management.

CLINICS CARE POINTS

- Historically, only 15% of patients with thoracic vascular injuries from blunt trauma make it to the hospital for definitive treatment.
- Pulse deficits are the most likely indication on sideline exam that there is a significant injury to the vasculature.
- POCUS can be an additional tool to help determine injury if available and there is appropriate operator experience.
- Blood pressure should be managed in the pre-hospital setting if hypertension is present.
- CT angiography should be obtained if there is concern for vascular injury.
- Surgery is the mainstay of definitive treatment.

CARDIAC INJURY
Introduction

Blunt cardiac injuries (BCI) encompass a wide range of pathologies, from clinically asymptomatic to fatal cardiac wall rupture. Among diagnosed BCIs, the most frequent diagnosis is "myocardial/cardiac contusion".[38] This type of injury occurs as a result of sudden deceleration or compression of the chest, such as in a motor vehicle accident or in contact and high-impact sports like football, hockey, MMA, or rugby.

Patient Evaluation Overview

The incidence of cardiac injury secondary to blunt chest trauma varies considerably,[39,40] as there is currently no accepted gold standard diagnostic test or diagnostic criteria. This lack of consensus makes diagnosing BCI challenging. History and physical exam suggestive of high-impact mechanism of injury should raise clinical suspicion. Patients may present with chest pain, dyspnea, palpitations, or presyncope. Other physical findings that may indicate BCI include tachypnea, irregular lung sounds, chest wall tenderness, chest abrasions or ecchymosis, rib, or sternal fractures. However, these findings are not specific to BCI and severe injuries in other areas may mask or distract from BCI symptoms.

The EAST published BCI practice guidelines in 2012, recommending an ECG for all suspected BCI cases.[41] Patients with abnormal ECG findings should be admitted for continuous cardiac monitoring. Sinus tachycardia is the most common dysrhythmia in BCI. Other dysrhythmias include new bundle branch blocks and ST or T wave abnormalities.[38] However, tachycardia in trauma patients should raise suspicion of ongoing bleeding rather than BCI. Once bleeding is ruled out, BCI becomes more likely in the differential diagnosis.

The utility of cardiac biomarkers in the setting of BCI is not well understood. Serial biomarkers should be measured in blunt thoracic trauma patients with evidence of ischemia or new conduction abnormalities, along with immediate consultation with both cardiology and cardiac surgery.[41] Nevertheless, negative troponins cannot exclude BCI or further complications, especially in the setting of significant ECG changes. Conversely, elevated troponins in a stable patient, without signs of severe injury or ECG abnormalities, have variable sensitivity and specificity for myocardial contusion and provide limited prognostic value.[41] Therefore, if concern exists, admission for brief observation with repeat physical exams, serial ECGs, and telemetry is preferable, as certain BCIs may have a delayed presentation.

Although not directly evaluating for cardiac contusion, plain radiographs should be obtained to evaluate for sternal or rib fractures, and pneumothorax, which correlate with high kinetic energy at impact.

Although CT, magnetic resonance imaging (MRI) and echocardiogram are not part of the initial diagnostic evaluation for BCI,[39] they can be complementary or useful in symptomatic patients without a clear clinical etiology and can be considered on a case-by-case basis though are often obtained given the overlap between mechanism and concern for additional injuries.

Medical Treatment Options

Given the wide range of presentations, the approach to managing cardiac contusions will depend on the severity of the injury and the presence of concurrent injuries.

If the mechanism of injury and clinical presentation are concerning for cardiac contusion, patients should generally be monitored with ECG and hemodynamic observation.[42] Although there are no established criteria for a monitoring time frame, 24 to 48 hours is reasonable for otherwise stable patients, as cardiac failure and most serious ventricular arrhythmias seldom present after this period.[39]

For patients with mild to moderate cardiac contusions, management is generally supportive, focusing on pain management and close monitoring for potential complications. Analgesics and anti-inflammatory medications may be used to manage pain and reduce inflammation.

Patients who develop new arrhythmias (including persistent tachycardia), signs of heart failure, or exhibit hemodynamic instability indicative of cardiac dysfunction, require cardiology consultation. The subset of patients with isolated abnormal ECG and/or cardiac biomarker elevations often has a benign course with rare long-term functional impairment.[42] Management of dysrhythmias should follow the same approach as for non-BCI patients: repleting electrolytes, avoiding hypoxia and acidosis, and utilizing anti-dysrhythmics along with advanced life support algorithms when clinically indicated.[28] Complete heart block may necessitate a pacemaker, although it is rare with isolated BCI. ST segment elevations may indicate either a contused heart or a traumatic myocardial infarction, requiring coronary angiography.[38]

For patients with minor ECG abnormalities, such as intermittent premature ventricular or atrial contractions, and normal hemodynamics, floor telemetry is appropriate.[39] Patients with significant dysrhythmias may require the intensive care unit. If arrhythmias persist during monitoring, a cardiology consultation should be obtained.

In more severe cases of cardiac contusions, surgical intervention may be necessary. In cases of cardiac tamponade, pericardiocentesis may be performed to remove fluid from the pericardial sac and relieve pressure on the heart. Rarely, surgical exploration and repair of cardiac injuries may be required.[38]

Evaluation of Outcome and/or Long-Term Recommendations

The prognosis of BCI depends on the type of cardiac injury, concurrent injuries, and the patient's history of previous cardiac disease or cardiac risk factors. Patients with isolated BCI and abnormal ECG or troponin levels tend to have a better outcome than those with hemodynamic compromise and cardiac structural injury with a high trauma injury score.[39] As the former group is more common, BCI generally has an overall favorable prognosis.

Immediate management is required for acute complications resulting from severe cardiac injuries, with long-term sequelae often arising from their specific injury. Although the majority of BCI patients do not experience long-term consequences, a few late complications have been documented, including delayed cardiac rupture, complete atrioventricular block, heart failure, pericardial effusion, and constrictive pericarditis.[39]

There are scarce data available to describe recovery times after a cardiac contusion. Based on the limited long-term outcome studies, patients diagnosed with myocardial contusions 6 and 12 months after an initial assessment showed normalization of all cardiac findings and no patient reported symptoms related to cardiac injury.[38,43]

Athletes with mild cardiac contusions may return to their sport after appropriate rest and medication within a few days to a couple of weeks, while more severe cardiac contusions can take several weeks to several months to heal.

SUMMARY/DISCUSSION/FUTURE DIRECTIONS

BCI is a challenging diagnosis due to its diverse presentation and spectrum of injury, coupled with the absence of a clear definition and diagnostic criteria. Nevertheless, high clinical suspicion for BCI is critical in trauma patients. Screening tools such as ECG and troponin levels can be used, followed by admission and echocardiography for any abnormalities, knowing that BCI may take up to 48 hours to manifest.

Although most BCI diagnoses may be inconsequential, the true significance of the diagnosis remains disputed due to the insufficient evaluation of long-term outcomes. Further consensus and research among health care providers are necessary to improve the definition and management of BCI and its long-term implications.

CLINICS CARE POINTS

- In otherwise healthy, hemodynamically stable patients with concern for isolated BCI, screening with serial ECGs, cardiac monitoring, and observation for 4 to 6 hours is sufficient.
- Life-threatening arrhythmias are managed with standard advanced cardiac life saving (ACLS) protocols, while structural damage requires immediate surgical consultation.
- There is no gold standard imaging modality for diagnosing BCI, however, a bedside FAST and/or formal echocardiogram should be considered in any patient with significant blunt thoracic trauma.

STERNOCLAVICULAR JOINT DISLOCATION
Introduction

Sternoclavicular (SC) joint dislocations are not a common injury, however, when they do occur, can be potentially life-threatening. SC joint dislocations account for only 1% of all traumatic joint dislocations[44] and make up only 3% of all shoulder dislocations.[45]

The SC joint serves as the only bony articulation between the axial skeleton and the upper extremity. Dislocation of this joint most commonly occurs due to a high-energy trauma. Many sports involve high-energy trauma to the chest region, making this rare injury one that may occur with higher frequency in the athletic population. The SC joint can dislocate either anteriorly or posteriorly, with a posterior dislocation raising more possible complications due to the underlying anatomy, including neurovascular bundles running to the head and neck, specifically the subclavian artery and vein, brachial plexus, vagus nerve, recurrent laryngeal nerve, as well as the trachea, esophagus, larynx, and lung.

Patient Evaluation Overview

These patients will present most commonly after a high-energy traumatic mechanism. Typically, they will complain of proximal to mid-clavicular pain. Anterior dislocations typically present with a painful lump at the SC joint. Depending on the mechanism of injury, it may be difficult to distinguish a true anterior dislocation from a medial clavicular fracture. In patients with posterior dislocations, there may be only mild to no swelling, and may have a small depression in the location of the SC joint.[45] The arm is often held in adduction for stability.

Patients need to be immediately evaluated for any neurovascular changes or deficits. These include, but are not limited to, dyspnea, phonation changes, dysphagia, venous congestion, neurologic deficits in the affected arm, and any stroke symptoms.[44] If any of these findings are present, the dislocation should be reduced as quickly as possible.

Once SC joint dislocation is determined to be the most likely diagnosis, imaging should be obtained. Plain films are the first step, but unfortunately, they lack sensitivity. They do provide additional information about underlying structures and complications such as pneumothorax, location of trachea, etc. Both the Serendipity view (**Fig. 1**) and the Heinig view have been used to identify an SC dislocation.[46] Due to the poor sensitivity of x-ray, CT scan (**Fig. 2.**) is typically the standard for diagnosis.

Pharmacologic or Medical Treatment Options

For posterior dislocations, there are no great options for medical management alone. Pain control will be key for reduction, but all posterior dislocations should be reduced.[47]

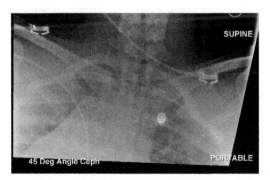

Fig. 1. Serendipity view of the clavicle in a patient with a left posterior SC joint dislocation. Images are the author's (Alex Tomesch, MD).

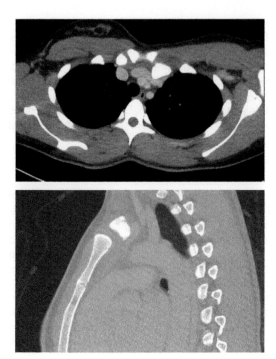

Fig. 2. Axial and sagittal CT imaging shows left posterior dislocation of the SC joint with compression of the subclavian vein. Images are the author's own (Alex Tomesch, MD).

Anterior dislocations initially were treated conservatively without reduction, but in follow-up studies, there have been many complications from conservative treatment including decreased function, pain with activity, and post-traumatic arthritis.[48] Therefore, these are ideally treated with reduction as well.

Non-Pharmacologic or Surgical/Interventional Treatment Options

Both anterior and posterior SC joint dislocations should be managed with reduction. Closed reduction should be attempted first, however, the success rate is not exceedingly high (38%).[49] Oftentimes, these reductions will take place in the operating room (OR) under general anesthesia and intubated status.

Posterior Dislocations: With the patient supine, a bolster should be placed under the scapula to allow for shoulder extension, abduction, and extension of the ipsilateral arm with anteroposterior pressure applied on bilateral shoulders and concomitant traction to the ipsilateral arm is the technique that can be used.[47] Additionally, a towel clip can be used to grasp the medial clavicle and pull it anteriorly.[45]

Anterior Dislocations: With the patient supine, a bolster should be placed between the shoulders. Traction is applied to the ipsilateral arm in 90 degrees of abduction with neutral flexion. Then, direct anteroposterior pressure is applied over the medial clavicle.[45] If closed reduction is unsuccessful, open reduction and internal fixation are not well described and most often will likely be treated non-operatively. In a high-level athlete or high-functioning young patient, an open reduction with internal fixation (ORIF) may be considered.[44]

Combination Therapies

None.

Treatment Resistance/Complications

When considering anterior SC joint injury, it is important to rule out fractures in patients who are under the age of 25. The medial physis of the clavicle is the last physis to close and therefore is at risk of injury.[44–47,49,50] Therefore, some anterior SC joint presentations may appear to be dislocations but could be fractures through the physis.

As outlined above, there are many potential complications of posterior SC joint dislocation including and up to death (3%–4% of injuries).[46] Surgeries have historically been performed with cardiothoracic surgery present and available due to the significant structures involved posterior to the SC joint.

New Developments

Historically, most interventions are performed in the OR with cardiothoracic surgery available due to the high stakes and potential for injury to surrounding structures. However, a recent meta-analysis[44] does note that no injuries to the surrounding structures have been reported before their publication (2019), and they suggest that cardiothoracic surgery may not need to always be involved.

Evaluation of Outcome and/or Long-Term Recommendations

Posterior Dislocation: A review of open reductions shows that 10% to 20% of patients have complications with continued pain, and decreased physical activity/function. Most of these studies followed these patients for 1 to 3 years.

Anterior Dislocation: If unable to reduce the dislocation non-operatively, there are risks for prolonged pain, arthritis, and decreased mobility, however, there are not any currently proven techniques. Therefore, if they are not high-functioning, relatively young individuals, leaving it unreduced is likely the best option.

SUMMARY/DISCUSSION/FUTURE DIRECTIONS

Overall, SC joint dislocation can be a serious problem, particularly posterior dislocations. These patients need to have a thorough evaluation on the sideline and be taken to a local hospital for evaluation if there is a concern for SC injury. CT scan is the gold standard of diagnosis and can provide additional information about other involved structures. Many of these injuries will end up requiring surgical intervention, with non-operative reduction only having a 38% success rate. Having the patient in a controlled environment like the OR is best before attempting reduction if there are no life-threatening associated injuries requiring emergent intervention.

CLINICS CARE POINTS

- SC joint dislocations are very uncommon but can be potentially life-threatening injuries.
  - They account for only 1% of all traumatic joint dislocations[44] and make up only 3% of all shoulder dislocations.[45]
- Symptoms are typically medial clavicular pain and/or deformity.
- If there are signs of dyspnea, phonation changes, dysphagia, venous congestion, neurologic deficits in the affected arm, and for any stroke symptoms,[44] consider rapid or urgent intervention with reduction.

- If there are not any symptoms of compression of significant structures, reduction in a controlled setting such as an OR is recommended.
- Consider having cardiothoracic surgery available before intervention.
  - However, there have not been any reports of required cardiothoracic intervention after reduction.
- Return to activity is often prolonged, however, most patients are able to return to previous levels of activity.

DISCLOSURE

The Authors have nothing to disclose.

REFERENCES

1. Sherwood DH, Gill BD, Schuessler BA, et al. Posttraumatic pneumothorax in sport: a case report and management algorithm. Curr Sports Med Rep 2021; 20(3):133–6.
2. Feden JP. Closed lung trauma. Clin Sports Med 2013;32(2):255–65.
3. Partridge RA, Coley A, Bowie R, et al. Sports-related pneumothorax. Ann Emerg Med 1997;30(4):539–41.
4. Sharma A, Jindal P. Principles of diagnosis and management of traumatic pneumothorax. J Emerg Trauma Shock 2008;1(1):34–41.
5. Wilkerson RG, Stone MB. Sensitivity of bedside ultrasound and supine anteroposterior chest radiographs for the identification of pneumothorax after blunt trauma. Acad Emerg Med 2010;17(1):11–7.
6. Wernick B, Hon HH, Mubang RN, et al. Complications of needle thoracostomy: a comprehensive clinical review. Int J Crit Illn Inj Sci. 2015;5(3):160–9.
7. Bunch A, Duchateau FX, Verner L, et al. Commercial air travel after pneumothorax: a review of the literature. Air Med J 2013;32(5):268–74.
8. Takada K, Matsumoto S, Hiramatsu T, et al. Spontaneous pneumomediastinum: an algorithm for diagnosis and management. Ther Adv Respir Dis 2009;3(6): 301–7.
9. Olson RP. Return to collision sport after pneumomediastinum. Curr Sports Med Rep 2012;11(2):58–63.
10. Esayag Y, Furer V, Izbicki G. Spontaneous pneumomediastinum: is a chest X-ray enough? A single-center case series. Isr Med Assoc J 2008;10(8–9):575–8.
11. Chaudhary H, Yousaf Z, Nasir U, et al. Spontaneous pneumomediastinum mimicking acute pericarditis. Clin Case Rep 2021;9(12):e05156.
12. Szymanski TJ, Jaklitsch MT, Jacobson F, et al. Expansion of postoperative pneumothorax and pneumomediastinum: determining when it is safe to fly. Aviat Space Environ Med 2010;81(4):423–6.
13. Tobushi T, Hosokawa K, Matsumoto K, et al. Exercise-induced pneumomediastinum. Int J Emerg Med 2015;8(1):43.
14. Leiber MJ, Phan NT. Pneumomediastinum and subcutaneous emphysema in a synchronized swimmer. Phys Sportsmed 2005;33(8):40–3.
15. Dyste KH, Newkirk KM. Pneumomediastinum in a high school football player: a case report. J Athl Train 1998;33(4):362–4.
16. Zarandy E, Counts S, Clemow C. Pneumomediastinum in a college-aged soccer player: a case report. Curr Sports Med Rep 2017;16(2):71–3.
17. Perez J, Teatino R. Pneumomediastinum in a snorkeling diver. BMJ Case Rep 2012;2012. https://doi.org/10.1136/bcr.09.2011.4776. bcr0920114776.

18. Gregory PL, Biswas AC, Batt ME. Musculoskeletal problems of the chest wall in athletes. Sports Med 2002;32(4):235–50.

19. Rainer TH, Griffith JF, Lam E, et al. Comparison of thoracic ultrasound, clinical acumen, and radiography in patients with minor chest injury. J Trauma 2004; 56(6):1211–3.

20. Yang Y, Young JB, Schermer CR, et al. Use of ketorolac is associated with decreased pneumonia following rib fractures. Am J Surg 2014;207(4):566–72.

21. Burton SW, Riojas C, Gesin G, et al. Multimodal analgesia reduces opioid requirements in trauma patients with rib fractures. J Trauma Acute Care Surg 2022;92(3): 588–96.

22. Kring RM, Mackenzie DC, Wilson CN, et al. Ultrasound-guided serratus anterior plane block (SAPB) improves pain control in patients with rib fractures. J Ultrasound Med 2022;41(11):2695–701.

23. Surdhar I, Jelic T. The erector spinae plane block for acute pain management in emergency department patients with rib fractures. CJEM 2022;24(1):50–4.

24. Akça AH, Şaşmaz Mİ, Kaplan Ş. Kinesiotaping for isolated rib fractures in emergency department. Am J Emerg Med 2020;38(3):638–40.

25. Quick G. A randomized clinical trial of rib belts for simple fractures. Am J Emerg Med 1990;8(4):277–81.

26. Dwyer MK, Uhl TL. A traumatic pneumothorax as a result of a rib fracture in a college baseball player. Orthopedics 2003;26(7):726–7.

27. Marco CA, Sorensen D, Hardman C, et al. Risk factors for pneumonia following rib fractures. Am J Emerg Med 2020;38(3):610–2.

28. Omori K, Jitsuiki K, Majima T, et al. Aortic injury due to paragliding: a case reporT. Int J Sports Phys Ther 2017;12(3):390–401.

29. Mayerick C, Carré F, Elefteriades J. Aortic dissection and sport: physiologic and clinical understanding provide an opportunity to save young lives. J Cardiovasc Surg 2010;51(5):669–81.

30. Hatzaras I, Tranquilli M, Coady M, et al. Weight lifting and aortic dissection: more evidence for a connection. Cardiology 2007;107(2):103–6.

31. Singhal P, Kejriwal N. Ascending aortic tear with severe aortic regurgitation following rugby injury. Heart Lung Circ 2009;18(2):150–1.

32. Heller G, Immer FF, Savolainen H, et al. Aortic rupture in high-speed skiing crashes. J Trauma 2006;61(4):979–80.

33. Haber R, Weisz GM. Contact sport-induced coronary artery dissection. Isr Med Assoc J 2019;21(8):555–6.

34. O'Conor CE. Diagnosing traumatic rupture of the thoracic aorta in the emergency department. Emerg Med J 2004;21(4):414–9.

35. Fox N, Schwartz D, Salazar JH, et al. Evaluation and management of blunt traumatic aortic injury: a practice management guideline from the Eastern Association for the Surgery of Trauma. J Trauma Acute Care Surg 2015;78(1):136–46, published correction appears in J Trauma Acute Care Surg. 2015 Feb;78(2):447.

36. Sturm JT, Marsh DG, Kenton CB. Ruptured thoracic aorta: evolving radiological concepts. Surgery 1987;85:363–7.

37. Babu GG, Wood A, O'Callaghan P, et al. The complete array of electrocardiogram abnormalities secondary to myocardial contusion in a single case. Europace 2009;11(11):1557–9.

38. Gunnar WP, Martin M, Smith RF, et al. The utility of cardiac evaluation in the hemodynamically stable patient with suspected myocardial contusion. Am Surg 1991;57:373–7.

39. Nair L, Winkle B, Senanayake E, et al. Managing Blunt Cardiac Injury. J Cardiothorac Surg 2023;18(1). https://doi.org/10.1186/s13019-023-02146-z.

40. Singh S, Heard M, Pester JM, et al. Blunt Cardiac Injury. In: StatPearls. Treasure Island (FL): StatPearls Publishing, 28, October, 2022.

41. Collins JN, Cole FJ, Weireter LJ, et al. The usefulness of serum troponin levels in evaluating cardiac injury. Am Surg 2001;67(9):821–6.

42. Clancy K, Velopulos C, Bilaniuk J, et al. Screening for blunt cardiac injury. J Trauma Acute Care Surg 2012;73(5). https://doi.org/10.1097/ta.0b013e318270193a.

43. Sturaitis M, McCallum D, Sutherland G, et al. Lack of significant long-term sequelae following traumatic myocardial contusion. Arch Intern Med 1986;146: 1765–9.

44. Sernandez H, Riehl J. Sternoclavicular joint dislocation: a systematic review and meta-analysis. J Orthop Trauma 2019;33(7):e251–5.

45. Morell DJ, Thyagarajan DS. Sternoclavicular joint dislocation and its management: a review of the literature. World J Orthop 2016;7(4):244–50.

46. Sewell MD, Al-Hadithy N, Le Leu A, et al. Instability of the sternoclavicular joint: current concepts in classification, treatment and outcomes. Bone Joint Lett J 2013;95-B:721–31.

47. Deren ME, Behrens SB, Vopat BG, et al. Posterior sternoclavicular dislocations: a brief review and technique for closed management of a rare but serious injury. Orthop Rev 2014;6(1). https://doi.org/10.4081/or.2014.5245.

48. de Jong KP, Kaulesar Sukul DMKS. Anterior sternoclavicular dislocation: a long-term follow-up study. J Orthop Trauma 1990;4(4):420–3.

49. Groh GI, Wirth MA, Rockwood CA Jr. Treatment of traumatic posterior sternoclavicular dislocations. J Shoulder Elbow Surg 2011;20(1):107–13.

50. Glass ER, Thompson JD, Cole PA, et al. Treatment of sternoclavicular joint dislocations: a systematic review of 251 dislocations in 24 case series. J Trauma Inj Infect Crit Care 2011;70(5):1294–8.

Acute Hemorrhage on the Playing Field

Alecia Gende, DO, CAQSM[a,b,]*, Heather Roesly, MD, CAQSM[c,d]

KEYWORDS

- Hemorrhage • Bleeding • Hemostasis • Tourniquet • Trauma

KEY POINTS

- Hemostasis is the mainstay of managing hemorrhage on the playing field.
- Direct pressure and in certain situations, tourniquet use or use of hemostatic topical agents and bandages are fast and safe methods to achieve hemostasis.
- Fracture stabilization with splinting or pelvic binders may assist with significant hemorrhage control in fractures of the pelvis or femur.
- Activation of the emergency action plan is necessary with any major or uncontrollable bleeding or with high clinical suspicion for internal bleeding.
- Universal precautions when possible while caring for bleeding athletes.

INTRODUCTION

Acute injury with bleeding occurs when blunt or penetrating trauma causes blood vessel damage. Acute hemorrhage can range in severity dependent on the type of blood vessel damage, leading to the loss of athlete participation, infection, and in more severe cases can threaten life or limb. Given the wide range in severity of acute hemorrhage and its frequency in sport, identification and management of bleeding on the playing field are critical skills for sideline sports medicine professionals. Recognizing and addressing hemorrhage early can decrease infection risk, allow for faster return to play, and improve morbidity and mortality outcomes for athletes on the field.

This article addresses various types of wounds and vessel bleeding, early identification of acute hemorrhage, and sideline management options for controlling hemorrhage on the playing field. The authors discuss types of hemorrhage, common injuries that lead to hemorrhage, and strategies to achieve hemostasis before athlete return to play or transport.

---

[a] Department of Emergency Medicine, Mayo Clinic Health System, 700 West Avenue, La Crosse, WI 54601, USA; [b] Department of Sports Medicine, Mayo Clinic Health System, 700 West Avenue, La Crosse, WI 54601, USA; [c] Emergency Medicine Faculty, University of Colorado, Aurora, CO, USA; [d] UC Health Highlands Ranch Hospital, 1500 Central Drive, Highlands Ranch, CO 80129-6688, USA
* Corresponding author. 700 West Avenue, La Crosse, WI 54601.
E-mail address: gende.alecia@mayo.edu

Clin Sports Med 42 (2023) 401–408
https://doi.org/10.1016/j.csm.2023.02.005
0278-5919/23/© 2023 Elsevier Inc. All rights reserved.

sportsmed.theclinics.com

PATIENT EVALUATION

Prompt and accurate recognition of different types and the severity of hemorrhage is a crucial skill for sideline professionals as it guides early management of common minor and major injuries. Small vessel bleeding is less likely to lead to life or limb threat and can often be managed easily on the sideline, whereas large vessel bleeding is more difficult to manage and may require application of emergent adjuncts or pharmaceuticals to achieve hemostasis.

TYPES OF ACUTE HEMORRHAGE

Capillary bleeding:
- Most common example is abrasions or scrapes
- Seen also with subconjunctival hemorrhage
- May also manifest as petechiae or bruising

Venous Bleeding:
- Common examples are lacerations, puncture wounds to extremities
- Internal bleeding, pelvis, abdomen and solid organs are potential sites
- Epistaxis is most commonly venous bleeding

Arterial Bleeding
- Common examples are lacerations to extremities, either in locations where arteries are superficial or with deeper lacerations
- Consider arterial bleeding with amputations and with extremity or pelvis fractures
- Penetrating chest trauma may be a combination of arterial and venous bleeding

RECOGNITION OF BLEEDING

When evaluating patients, signs of external bleeding may be straight forward. The direct visualization of bleeding from a wound, whether capillary, venous, or arterial, is relatively easy to identify. However, identifying those at risk for and the clinical signs of internal bleeding can be more subtle and may require repeated examinations. The most important aspect of identification of internal bleeding is maintaining a high level of suspicion, especially in sport-specific scenarios.

Acute internal hemorrhage is most common in high-velocity blunt trauma. Beyond contact or combat sports, maintain a high clinical suspicion in athletes traveling at higher speeds or participating in downhill events such as skiing or cycling and consider in athletes falling from a height such as those involved in jumping sports, ski jumping, water skiing, or sky diving. Always keep internal hemorrhage in the differential diagnosis for athletes injured traveling on motorized or higher speed vehicles, such as motocross, motorcycle, and snowmobile racing. Although only a few scenarios are mentioned here, it is important to consider the risk of athletes in each sport to be adequately prepared.

Internal bleeding can occur in the major cavities of the body including the head, chest, abdomen, pelvis, or compartments of the extremity. Because athletes are generally healthy, they may be able to mask the early signs of bleeding. Monitoring and frequent assessments of athletes after a high-risk or dangerous mechanism of injury are important and can be life-saving.

Although signs of internal bleeding are frequently subtle, continued bleeding can produce signs of hemorrhagic shock. It is imperative to be vigilant for signs of shock during the post-traumatic monitoring period. These include decreasing alertness, lightheadedness, pallor, and diaphoresis as well as changes in vital signs. As stated, in the early stages of hemorrhagic shock, many athletes may compensate quite well and have normal vital signs. However, as blood loss continues and hemorrhagic shock progresses, athletes will generally develop a tachycardia and eventually hypotension.[1] These signs should increase suspicion for internal bleeding, usually into the larger cavities of the body including the chest, abdomen, pelvis, or thigh and lead to prompt activation of the emergency action plan (EAP) and notification of emergency medical services.

If vital sign abnormalities are assessed, a sideline evaluation of the chest, abdomen, pelvis, and thighs should be performed to help guide immediate management as EAP is activated. Bruising or deformity to the abdomen or chest wall may indicate a severe internal injury that requires urgent transport to the nearest hospital or trauma center for more definitive management. Depending on the personal level of skill, a mobile ultrasound may be used to confirm the presence of internal bleeding. Point-of-care ultrasound, specifically focused assessment with sonography in trauma (FAST), can be quickly assessed and if positive should lead to prompt evacuation of athlete to nearest trauma center for emergent care. A negative or normal FAST examination can be reassuring but does not definitively rule out internal hemorrhage. Literature demonstrates the sensitivity of FAST examination ranging from 85% to 96% and specificity from 98% to 100%.[2] As stated, a negative FAST examination cannot independently rule out internal bleeding, but a positive FAST examination can assist in prompt identification of intra-abdominal hemorrhage and activation of EAP.

Fractures are another cause of significant bleeding. Open fractures and severely displaced fractures may produce an obvious source and degree of noticeable hemorrhage in the athlete. Thigh deformities and leg shortening should increase clinical suspicion for femur fractures. A fractured femur can lacerate veins and arteries in the thigh and lead to bleeding into the thigh compartments. Femur fractures may require reduction and stabilization with a splint to help minimize bleeding. Occasionally, a tourniquet may be required to control extremity hemorrhage. This is more thoroughly discussed in the next section.

Potentially more difficult to assess, pelvic fractures can lacerate internal pelvic blood vessels, veins, and/or arteries and can lead to life-threatening bleeding. Pelvic instability can be assessed by feeling movement or laxity with a compression of the hips. If present, a high index of suspicion for a pelvic fracture should be maintained and the sports medicine professional should take action to control hemorrhage and active the EAP. Unfortunately, physical examination to evaluate for pelvic fractures is unreliable and may even lead to more bleeding; therefore, one must have a high index of suspicion based on the mechanism of injury.[3,4] In a more alert athlete, the presence of groin, hip, or back pain should increase concerns for pelvic fracture and hemorrhage. When an athlete has a depressed level of alertness, the mechanism of injury should direct providers to consider pelvic fractures and hemorrhage as a potential injury. The prehospital management of pelvic hemorrhage is direct compression and fracture stabilization, usually with a pelvic binder, placed over the greater trochanters, which serves as a source of circumferential compression to the broken pelvis and injured blood vessels.[4,5] A variety of commercial made binders exist.

Noticing signs of internal bleeding, vital sign abnormalities, altered level of consciousness, and high-risk injury patterns should prompt sideline professionals to trigger the EAP for evacuation and consideration of emergency adjuncts such as pelvic binders, fracture reduction and traction splinting, and tourniquet use when appropriate.

MANAGEMENT OF BLEEDING

The primary objective in addressing all types of bleeding is hemostasis. Hemostasis occurs naturally in the body via a complex cascade that involves clot formation along an injured vessel. Hemostasis occurs when a temporary platelet clot forms on the injured vessel. Eventually, a sturdier and more robust fibrin clot reinforces this temporary clot to prevent rebleeding and allow the healing process to take place at the site of injury. This can be more rapidly achieved in an emergent situation using direct pressure, cautery, and topical or systemic medications. These interventions are geared toward aiding the hemostasis pathway by either allowing for more rapid vasoconstriction, formation of a platelet clot, formation of a fibrin clot, or in preventing the breakdown of clot products. Given the limitations of on-field and sideline management, the authors focus our discussion on direct pressure application and topical pharmacologic medications.

PHARMACOLOGIC VERSUS NON-PHARMACOLOGIC BLEEDING MANAGEMENT

On the sideline, hemorrhage management should be focused on return to play, stabilization, and/or transport. By far and large, the staples of hemostasis revolve around the use of pressure. The application of direct pressure can help to control the majority of bleeding events from capillaries, veins, and even arteries. The application of direct pressure should be firm and constant, which allows a platelet plug to form on the injured vessel and is interrupted any time pressure is let up. The direct pressure application may be required for several minutes for the natural process to successfully occur. When possible, applying direct pressure with a smaller surface area, such as a finger applied to the source of bleeding, is more beneficial than using a larger surface area such as the palm of a hand or a pressure dressing. This allows the force of pressure to be focused on the source of bleeding rather than distributed equally among the bleeding source and the surrounding area. This is especially helpful to consider when dealing with higher pressure bleeding, such as bleeding from arterial injuries. Emergency adjuncts such as pelvic binders, pressure dressings, and tourniquets all rely on the principles of direct pressure application. These adjuncts help to apply forces greater than sideline professionals and allow for direct and constant pressure application, whereas the medical professional's hands are free for other assessments and interventions.

There are some cases where bleeding can be more difficult to control, especially given time constraints in some sports for return to play. In these particular cases, topical medications are beneficial when used along with direct pressure application to more definitively and rapidly stop bleeding. This is frequently the case with epistaxis, common to boxing, wrestling, and combat sports. The classic progression of epistaxis management during competition or practice involves constant, direct pressure with a nasal clamp, if bleeding is not controlled, the sideline professional will advance quickly to topical agents such as oxymetazoline or others discussed below and may further advance with direct pressure via nasal packing.[6]

PHARMACOLOGICS
Oxymetazoline

Oxymetazoline is an alpha-1 and alpha-2 agonist which leads to blood vessel constriction. This tends to work best when applied to small bleeding veins (such as those in the nose) which can help to aid in rapid termination of epistaxis, especially when used with direct pressure application. It is over the counter and can be purchased in a small container with an aerosolizing cap to allow for quick administration and is generally easy to store in a medical supply bag along with alternative non-pharmacologic tools to help with bleeding or epistaxis.

Tranexamic Acid

Tranexamic acid (TXA) is an antifibrinolytic medication than inhibits the breakdown of plasminogen and fibrin. This essentially prevents clot breakdown and allows for the formation of a more stable, faster forming clot which assists to slow down bleeding. This medication can be used systemically or topically but would generally be best for sideline use topically. TXA comes as a solvent which can be applied to gauze or packing and placed at the site of bleeding. TXA has been shown to be 3.5 times more effective in achieving hemostasis when applied with direct pressure for treatment of epistaxis.[7]

Hemostatic Dressings

Various hemostatic dressings use pharmacologic means to assist with clot formation and hemostasis. They work by two main mechanisms: formation of adhesive bandage or agent that covers the wound and activation of clotting factors to stimulate the natural clotting process. Surgicel is a plant-based cellulose polymer dressing that is absorbable when exposed to moisture, such as a bleeding wound. Its absorption by the body creates a temporary coagulation of blood which can serve as a temporary clot, whereas the body's natural hemostasis cascade takes effect.[8] Surgicel can be placed as the first layer for many pressure dressings and can help allow for early hemostasis. QuikClot, occasionally referred to as Combat Gauze, is another hemostatic bandage. It is a kaolin-impregnated gauze that achieves hemostasis by initiating the coagulation cascade and accelerating clot formation. Various studies show quicker time to clot detection and less blood loss.[9,10]

NON-PHARMACOLOGICS
Wound Packing

Direct pressure for hemostatic control can be achieved with wound packing. Wound packing may consist of gauze in different forms, tampon or balloon packing. Nasal tampons and balloon packing are seen commonly in the case of persistent epistaxis. Various gauze dressings are packed directly into an extremity or abdominal wound and secured with further direct pressure. Dressings should be reinforced with an additional layer rather than removed and changed as needed for continued bleeding.

Tourniquet

Tourniquet use applies compression to proximal blood vessels thus limiting hemorrhage in extremity injury. Although in the past, use has been controversial and limited to the military population, current recommendations encourage tourniquet use and research has demonstrated minimal complications with use in civilian settings.[11–13] Proper tourniquet application involves placement generally, "high and tight" on the extremity but at least 2 to 3 inches proximal to the hemorrhaging wound.[14] The tourniquet should be tightened until distal bleeding ceases. A variety of commercial tourniquets are available, and most will offer a place to document time of placement for future providers information. The *Stop the Bleed* campaign is a national course for medical providers and lay people alike to aid in comfort and provide instruction for bleeding control and tourniquet placement.

Pelvic Binder

Prehospital management of pelvic hemorrhage is direct compression and fracture stabilization, usually with a pelvic binder which serves as a source of circumferential compression to the broken pelvis.[4,5] A variety of commercial made binders exist. There are case reports of using a bedsheet when a commercial binder is not available.[5] Pelvic binder application should be considered with any clinical suspicion for pelvic fractures based on the examination and mechanism of injury. One common mistake with pelvic binder placement is placement too high on the pelvis, over the iliac crests. Appropriate placement should be directed over the greater trochanters.

MANAGING DIFFERENT TYPES OF BLEEDING

Capillary bleeding:
- Pressure, cleansing, dressing
- May be promptly returned to play

Venous Bleeding:
- Direct pressure, pressure dressing, and hemostatic dressing
- Fracture or extremity management may require tourniquet use, secure "high and tight," at least 2 to 3 inches above the wound and avoid application directly onto a joint
- Pelvis vessel/fracture bleeding, circumferential pressure, and fracture stabilization with pelvic binder
- Epistaxis management direct pressure, pharmacologics, and nasal packing
- Based on hemostasis and sport, may tolerate safe return to play

Arterial Bleeding:
- Direct and constant pressure, focal versus generalized pressure when able
- Consider hemostatic dressing if available
- Tourniquet application, secure "high and tight," at least 2 to 3 inches above the wound and avoid application directly onto a joint
- Internal bleeding, lacerated artery secondary to fracture
- Consider traction splinting for femur fractures and pelvic binders for pelvis fractures
- Less likely to return to play on day of injury, more likely to require activation of EAP

Treatment Resistance

In the setting of extremity hemorrhage where direct pressure and wound packing is failing, the sideline professional may need to escalate care. This may involve use of more invasive nasal packing or topical hemostatic agents in epistaxis or escalation to a tourniquet in extremity hemorrhage. Tourniquet use should be considered promptly for obvious severe hemorrhage or arterial bleeding. Proper tourniquet placement is discussed in previous section. In some situations, a single tourniquet is unable to control bleeding. When this occurs, a second tourniquet is recommended with placement being even more proximal than the initial tourniquet. As a reminder, always document time of tourniquet placement and never remove a tourniquet once it has been placed. If unable to achieve hemostasis despite described measures, if tourniquet placement is required or if severe mechanism of injury, signs of shock or internal bleeding, prompt activation of the EAP is indicated and can be life-saving.

Evaluation of Outcome

Based on the severity of hemorrhage, once hemostasis is achieved the sideline professional should consider return to play or activation of EAP. With minor or controlled bleeding, such as minor lacerations, epistaxis, or abrasions, an athlete may promptly return to play after dressing application and hemostasis. However, repeat assessments are required and rebleeding may occur with return to play. More severe hemorrhage, uncontrollable hemorrhage or concern for internal bleeding should trigger EAP and reassessment until emergency medical services (EMS) arrival and transport.

Universal Precautions

Universal precautions refer to a set of guidelines introduced by the Centers for Disease Control to be used in any medical scenario, but particularly by health care providers to limit the spread of blood borne illnesses and infection.[15] Universal precautions should be considered by any sideline providers when dealing with acute hemorrhage or any time there is a potential exposure to blood or other bodily fluids (other than sweat). These emphasize the use of appropriate hand hygiene and personal protective equipment.

Whenever possible, sideline providers should practice appropriate hand hygiene before dealing with a bleeding wound.[16] Because of limited access to soap and water at most events, the use of portable hand sanitizer is appropriate. Any time, alcohol-based sanitizers are applied, and hands should be rubbed until dry. Hand hygiene should be practiced before coming in contact with wounds as well as after to limit spread of infection to both athletes and sideline providers.

Although personal protective equipment may be in short supply in some situations, it is important to always carry a set of gloves which can be easily accessed when dealing with wounds. Gloves act as an additional barrier of protection. They do not negate the need for appropriate hand sanitation whenever time allows.

Practicing sideline medicine is certainly different that providing care in a hospital or clinic and some situations may limit the ability to follow this set of guidelines, especially in emergent situations. Regardless, the use of hand sanitation and gloves can help limit infection risk to both athletes and caretakers and are generally easily accessible and quick to apply. At the minimum, these practices should be applied whenever possible when dealing with acute hemorrhage on the field.

Summary

Acute hemorrhage in sport is a common occurrence, which needs to be identified early and managed appropriately for the best outcomes in athletes. Sports medicine professionals need to understand the basics of acute hemorrhage care and have a standard approach to treating all wounds. This should include recognition of venous versus arterial bleeding, early recognition of internal hemorrhage, and should always include an emergency action plan for evacuation of athletes when necessary. Additional items such as pharmacologics including hemostatic dressings, dressings, and emergency adjuncts such as tourniquets and pelvic binders can be beneficial in the treatment of severe hemorrhage. These tools and this understanding will help sports medicine professionals safely and confidently care for the injured or bleeding athlete.

CLINICS CARE POINTS

- Universal precautions when possible
- Application of direct pressure first and foremost
- Tourniquet application, high and tight
  - Document time tourniquet places, never remove, always needs emergency action plan
- Pelvic binder in sport-specific and clinical scenarios where pelvic fracture is likely
- Traction splint in sport-specific scenarios and with obvious clinical signs of femur fracture
- If hemostasis achieved, always reevaluate to ensure continued hemostasis and no recurrence of bleeding

DISCLOSURE

The authors have nothing to disclose.

REFERENCES

1. Hooper N, Armstrong TJ. Hemorrhagic shock. (Updated 2022 Sep 26). In: Stat-Pearls (Internet). Treasure Island (FL): StatPearls Publishing; 2022. Available at: https://www.ncbi.nlm.nih.gov/books/NBK470382/.
2. Bloom BA, Gibbons RC. Focused assessment with sonography for trauma. [Updated 2022 Jul 25]. In: StatPearls [Internet]. Treasure Island (FL): StatPearls Publishing; 2022. Available at: https://www.ncbi.nlm.nih.gov/books/NBK470479/.
3. Okada Y, Nishioka N, Ohtsuru S, et al. Diagnostic accuracy of physical examination for detecting pelvic fractures among blunt trauma patients: a systematic review and meta-analysis. World J Emerg Surg 2020;15:56. https://doi.org/10.1186/s13017-020-00334-z.
4. Schweigkofler U, Wohlrath B, Trentsch H, et al. Diagnostics and early treatment in prehospital and emergency-room phase in suspicious pelvic ring fractures. Eur J Trauma Emerg Surg 2018;44(5):747–52.
5. Lee C, Porter K. The prehospital management of pelvic fractures. Emerg Med J 2007;24(2):130–3.
6. Womack JP, Kropa J, Jimenez Stabile M. Epistaxis: Outpatient Management. Am Fam Physician 2018;98(4):240–5.
7. Janapala RN, Tran QK, Patel J, et al. Efficacy of topical tranexamic acid in epistaxis: A systematic review and meta-analysis. Am J Emerg Med 2022;51:169–75.
8. Sileshi B, Achneck HE, Lawson JH. Management of surgical hemostasis: topical agents. Vascular 2008;16(Suppl 1). S22-8. Erratum in: Vascular. 2009;17(3):181.
9. Kheirabadi Bijan S, Scherer Michael RMA, Estep J Scot, et al. Determination of Efficacy of New Hemostatic Dressings in a Model of Extremity Arterial Hemorrhage in Swine. J Trauma: Injury, Infection, and Critical Care: September 2009; 67(3):450–60. https://doi.org/10.1097/TA.0b013e3181ac0c99.
10. Koko Kiavash RMD, McCauley Brian MMD, Gaughan John PPhD, et al. Kaolin-based hemostatic dressing improves hemorrhage control from a penetrating inferior vena cava injury in coagulopathic swine. J Trauma Acute Care Surg 2017; 83(1):71–6.
11. Beaucreux C, Vivien B, Miles E, et al. Application of tourniquet in civilian trauma: Systematic review of the literature. Anaesth Crit Care Pain Med 2018;37(6):597–606.
12. Smith AA, Ochoa JE, Wong S, et al. Prehospital tourniquet use in penetrating extremity trauma: Decreased blood transfusions and limb complications. J Trauma Acute Care Surg 2019;86(1):43–51.
13. Scerbo MH, Mumm JP, Gates K, et al. Safety and Appropriateness of Tourniquets in 105 Civilians. Prehosp Emerg Care 2016;20(6):712–22. https://doi.org/10.1080/10903127.2016.1182606.
14. Lei R, Swartz MD, Harvin JA, et al. Stop the Bleed Training empowers learners to act to prevent unnecessary hemorrhagic death. Am J Surg 2019;217(2):368–72.
15. Broussard IM, Kahwaji CI. Universal Precautions. [Updated 2022 Sep 1]. In: Stat-Pearls [Internet]. Treasure Island (FL): StatPearls Publishing; 2022.
16. Hoogenboom BJ, Smith D. Management of bleeding and open wounds in athletes. Int J Sports Phys Ther 2012;7(3):350–5.

Emergency Abdominopelvic Injuries

Ross E. Mathiasen, MD, CAQ-SM[a],*, Christopher P. Hogrefe, MD, CAQ-SM[b,c]

KEYWORDS

- Abdomen • Pelvic • Trauma • Sport • Return-to-play • Kidney • Liver • Spleen

KEY POINTS

- On the sideline, it is imperative to have a high clinical suspicion for abdominopelvic injuries to avoid a delay in definitive management.
- Any red flag signs or symptoms, particularly a worsening of pain more than time, should prompt an emergent evaluation (ie, in an emergency department).
- Computed tomography with intravenous contrast is the most sensitive imaging modality for acute abdominopelvic trauma.
- Return-to-play decisions should involve a multidisciplinary medical team (eg, general surgery, primary care, sports medicine, and so forth) given the absence of evidence-based guidelines.

INTRODUCTION

Sports-related abdominopelvic injuries have the potential to be catastrophic. At the time of first evaluation, these injuries may run the gamut from a relatively benign initial examination to hemorrhagic shock.[1] Therefore, clinicians must not only maintain a high index of suspicion for recognizing these maladies but also possess an understanding of the prehospital stabilization interventions, appropriate diagnostic modalities, and post-injury return-to-activity considerations.[2]

Most of the abdominopelvic injuries in sport are secondary to blunt trauma.[1,2] Contact sports serve as classic examples of potential mechanisms for such blunt abdominopelvic trauma (eg, football tackling, hockey checking); however, there are a multitude of other sports that place participants at risk for high-energy abdominopelvic trauma (eg, ski jumping, cycling, gymnastics).[1–5] Penetrating abdominal trauma,

[a] Department of Emergency Medicine, University of Nebraska Medical Center, 981150 Nebraska Medical Center, Omaha, NE 68198-1150, USA; [b] Department of Emergency Medicine, University of Iowa Hospitals and Clinics/University of Iowa Carver College of Medicine, 1008 RCP – 200 Hawkins Drive, Iowa City, IA 52242, USA; [c] Department of Orthopaedic Surgery, Northwestern Medicine/Northwestern University Feinberg School of Medicine, Chicago, IL, USA
* Corresponding author.
E-mail address: remathia@unmc.edu
Twitter: @chogrefe8 (C.P.H.)

Clin Sports Med 42 (2023) 409–425
https://doi.org/10.1016/j.csm.2023.02.006
0278-5919/23/© 2023 Elsevier Inc. All rights reserved.
sportsmed.theclinics.com

while exceedingly rare in sport, may also occur (eg, javelin, archery, high-impact skiing accidents).[6]

Overall, there is a paucity of evidence-based information related to abdominopelvic trauma in sport and associated recommendations for return-to-sport from these injuries. We present the clinical considerations regarding the evaluation and management of the most common traumatic abdominopelvic injuries in sport supported by the existing literature on the topics.

Differential Diagnosis

Based on the current research, the most frequently encountered abdominopelvic traumatic injuries in sport include liver laceration, splenic laceration, renal hematoma or laceration, rectus sheath hematoma, and hollow viscus injury to the intestine. Injuries to other organs within the abdominal and pelvic cavities may also occur, and thus, an understanding of the relevant anatomy is imperative to maintain a broad differential. Clinically, to aid in the diagnostic process the contents of the abdomen are often divided into quadrants. However, one must remember that some organs occupy multiple quadrants (eg, the large and small intestine, bladder, pancreas, and potentially the liver). In addition, some injuries may not reside within the abdominal cavity itself (eg, rectus sheath hematoma). Furthermore, the pelvic organs generally do not fall into this classification structure.

Within the right upper quadrant (RUQ) reside the liver (or the majority of it), gallbladder, pancreas (at least in part), right kidney, small intestine, and large intestine. The left upper quadrant (LUQ) contains the stomach, spleen, pancreas (at least a component thereof), left kidney, small intestine, and large intestine. The right lower quadrant (RLQ) contains the right ureter, small intestine, large intestine (including the appendix), and part of the bladder. The left lower quadrant contents are similar to the RLQ, with small intestine, large intestine, and a portion of the bladder. The pelvis itself may contain the right and left ovaries along with the uterus (if present). Other structures residing within the abdominopelvic cavity include the abdominal aorta and inferior vena cava. Several structures have minimal literature regarding traumatic injury in sport, specifically the stomach, gallbladder, ovaries, uterus, ureters, and aorta. Therefore, these organs are not reviewed further within this article.

CLINICAL FINDINGS
Patient Evaluation Overview

A high clinical suspicion for acute abdominopelvic injuries is imperative, as the initial presentation and examination may be benign at the time of injury. In fact, up to 50% of athletes with a significant intra-abdominal injury do not have red flags on initial physical examination (eg, peritonitis, hypotension, and hematuria). Up to 20% of athletes with hemoperitoneum (ie, blood within the peritoneum) may have an unremarkable early evaluation.[1]

The primary goal on the sideline or in the athletic training room should not be to diagnose a specific organ injury. Instead, the focus should be on identifying the signs and symptoms of acute pathology necessitating further evaluation and management followed by transportation of the athlete to the appropriate setting for continuation of care.[2] The emergency department is often the destination for these athletes as the definitive diagnosis of acute abdominopelvic trauma frequently necessitates laboratory analysis and advanced imaging modalities. In addition, management often consists of interventions that are not readily available on the sideline or in the athletic training room (eg, intravenous [IV] fluids, blood products, IV antibiotics, prolonged observation or hospitalization, embolization, surgery). In some instances, consulting services may be necessary (eg, interventional radiology, general surgery). Thus, the athlete should be transported whenever there is clinical concern for intra-abdominal pathology.[2,5,7,8]

When evaluating the injured athlete on the sideline, one should follow emergency medical protocols including performing a primary survey and activating the emergency action plan (EAP) as indicated. After the primary survey (ie, assessing the patient's airway, breathing, and circulation), the clinician may then proceed to a focused history and physical examination.[2,5] Regarding the pertinent history, it is imperative to appreciate the mechanism of injury, timing of the injury, current symptoms, and exacerbating and relieving factors. Obtaining a pertinent focused past medical history is also valuable when the clinical scenario allows. Items particularly relevant to abdominopelvic trauma include a history of previous abdominal surgeries or procedures, bleeding disorders, and use of anticoagulant medications.[8]

Red flags within the clinical history following acute abdominopelvic trauma include persistent or worsening abdominal pain, nausea or vomiting, hematuria, and pain radiating to the shoulder due to diaphragmatic irritation (ie, Kehr sign).[1,2,8] Examination red flags consist of tachycardia (or relative tachycardia in a well-conditioned athlete), decreased pulse volume (commonly described as a "thready pulse"), and hypotension.[1] Hypotension may be a late sign in pediatric patients or well-conditioned athletes and raises concern for significant blood loss.[6]

Visual inspection of the abdomen can be particularly revealing. Although "classic" findings may be present, their absence does not rule out acute intra-abdominal pathology. Several of these indicators may be delayed in their appearance surfacing days after the trauma. Periumbilical ecchymosis (Cullen's sign; **Fig. 1**), or bruising around the umbilicus, is typically associated with a pancreatic insult or pancreatitis. Gray Turner's sign (**Fig. 2**) is represented by bruising along the flanks or lateral aspect of the abdominal wall.[1,8,9] The presence of one of these signs raises concern for bleeding within the peritoneum or retroperitoneum (eg, splenic rupture).[1,8,9] A visible mass may also be present, raising concern for traumatic pathology (eg, a rectus sheath hematoma).

Palpation of the abdomen can assist in narrowing the differential diagnosis. Abdominal palpation should be performed with the patient in supine position. The abdominal examination is typically performed by palpating each abdominal quadrant. Tenderness within a specific quadrant increases suspicion that the injured structure lies within that quadrant. Tenderness may be present in multiple quadrants, which should raise concern for peritonitis (ie, inflammation or irritation of the lining of the abdominal

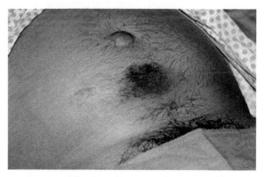

Fig. 1. Cullen's sign. (Cullen's sign, by Herbert L. Fred, MD and Hendrik A. van Dijk. https://commons.wikimedia.org/wiki/File:Cullen%27s_sign.jpg)

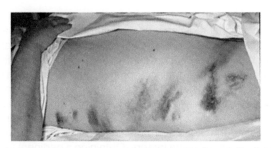

Fig. 2. Gray Turner's sign. (Hemorrhagic pancreatitis , by Herbert L. Fred, MD and Hendrik A. van Dijk. https://commons.wikimedia.org/wiki/Category:Grey_Turner%27s_sign#/media/File: Hemorrhagic_pancreatitis_-_Grey_Turner's_sign.jpg.)

cavity). Additional examination techniques to evaluate for peritonitis include evaluating for rebound or guarding. Rebound tenderness is the presence of pain when the examiner releases the manual pressure applied when palpating the abdomen and suggests the presence of peritonitis. Guarding, or flexing the abdominal musculature to decrease the pressure applied to the abdominal organs, should also increase suspicion for peritonitis. Meanwhile, an inability to lay flat for an abdominal examination secondary to abdominal pain is also concerning for peritonitis. Further assessment for peritonitis can include the heel tap sign, or raising the patient's leg approximately 20° off of the table and then tapping or hitting the bottom of the patient's heel with the examiner's free hand. A positive test entails causing abdominal pain when the heel is tapped, which suggests the presence of peritonitis.

A specific maneuver that can be valuable in differentiating between an abdominal musculature injury versus an intra-abdominal process is the Carnett sign. This sign entails first palpitating the point of maximal tenderness. Then, slightly lift the legs and torso of the patient off the examination surface, which contracts the abdominal musculature. If the pain remains the same or increases with palpation at the site of maximal tenderness, the injury is more likely to reside within the abdominal musculature (eg, ventral hernia). Otherwise, the abdominal examination may reveal a palpable mass. In the setting of acute trauma, a palpable mass should increase suspicion for the presence of a hematoma.

As previously noted, although the aforementioned findings may be readily apparent, the initial history and examination of the injured athlete with underlying abdominopelvic trauma may also be relatively benign. Thus, it is possible for a clinician to be faced with the delayed presentation of acute abdominopelvic traumatic pathology (eg, perforated hollow viscus).[2] In delayed presentations, the signs and symptoms of bacterial or chemical (eg, bile or blood) peritonitis may be present. Worsening abdominal pain more than time or a fever may indicate the development of peritonitis. Other indicators include abdominal pain exacerbated by minimal impact (eg, a car driving more than a bump in the road) and/or the presence of rebound or guarding on physical examination. These features should prompt the clinician to seek further investigation.

Although this article focuses on abdominopelvic trauma, it is imperative to remember that the original insult may involve another portion of the body (eg, thorax, back). For example, lower rib fractures may result in intra-abdominal injuries (eg, liver laceration). In addition, trauma to the back can similarly result in damage to intra-abdominal organs (eg, renal laceration). Consequently, the astute clinician should perform an abdominal examination in athletes reporting chest and/or back trauma.

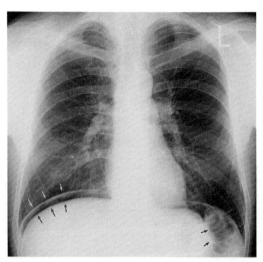

Fig. 3. Pneumoperitoneum on plain films (*Green arrows* represent the diaphragm; *red arrows* depict the liver edge; subdiaphragmatic air is noted between these regions; blue *arrows* highlight the cephalad migration of the intestines). (Pneumoperitoneum by Hellerhoff. https://commons.wikimedia.org/wiki/File:Pneumoperitoneum.jpg.)

Imaging Modalities

Abdominal plain films are not considered a first-line imaging modality for most intra-abdominal pathology. If abdominal plain films are secured to evaluate for free air in the abdomen (eg, bowel perforation) a lateral decubitus view should be included. Plain films have poor sensitivity for hollow viscus injury with less than 30% of patients with a visceral rupture having abnormal plain films (ie, pneumoperitoneum being visualized).[5] An abnormal study would show free air within the abdomen (**Fig. 3**). However, a normal study does not rule out pathology.[4,10] If one has concern for concomitant bony injury (eg, a pelvis fracture), plain films may be of utility in assessing these bony structures.[4]

Ultrasound (US) is frequently implemented in the emergency department and is increasingly used in the sideline setting for the evaluation of acute abdominopelvic trauma. The focused assessment with sonography in trauma (FAST) examination was developed for use in blunt trauma patients to evaluate for free intraperitoneal fluid (suggestive of bleeding) and for pericardial effusion, among other indications. This is a highly specific test (exceeding 98%) and an accurate screening tool (sensitivity 85% to 96%) that can be performed in less than 5 minutes.[1] The caveat of the sensitivity and sensitivity related to US being operator-dependent holds true, and thus its use requires appropriate equipment and training to be implemented successfully.[4]

The FAST examination entails obtaining images from four windows, specifically the cardiac, RUQ, LUQ, and suprapubic views (**Fig. 4**). Pertaining to intra-abdominal injury, the RUQ examination is abnormal if there is free fluid visualized within the hepatorenal recess (Morrison's pouch). On US, fluid appears black (or hypoechoic). The LUQ assessment is abnormal if there is fluid present within the perisplenic recess. Last, an abnormal suprapubic examination is reflected by free fluid in the retrovesicular space in males or retrouterine pouch in females (**Fig. 5**). In the sports medicine and sideline setting, the FAST examination may be used as a screening tool but not as a replacement for emergency department evaluation if clinical suspicion is high.

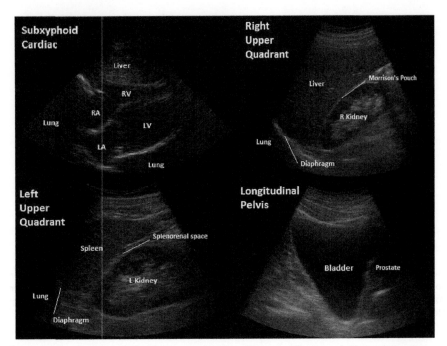

Fig. 4. Four windows of the FAST examination. (Trauma Ultrasound. From: https://www. nuemblog.com/trauma.)

Should there be clinical suspicion for an intra-abdominal injury in the setting of a negative FAST examination in a hemodynamically stable patient, further observation and/or workup is indicated, as the FAST examination may not reveal an intra-abdominal organ injury if no hemoperitoneum (or only a small volume hemoperitoneum) is present.[11] Further workup to consider in this clinical scenario includes a computed tomography (CT) with IV contrast, serial FAST examinations, and/or hospital observation monitoring for changes in clinical status and serial physical examinations.[11,12] In the emergency department setting, a positive FAST examination in a hemodynamically unstable patient is an indication for emergent surgical intervention.

CT with IV contrast remains the modality of choice for the evaluation of acute abdominopelvic trauma in hemodynamically stable patients. CT is more sensitive than other imaging options and enables injury grading (eg, liver laceration, spleen laceration).[1,4,8] If IV contrast is unable to be administered (eg, secondary to contrast allergy), a CT without contrast may have some utility in diagnosing large liver lacerations or hematoma. However, more subtle injuries (eg, small liver laceration, subcapsular splenic hematoma) may be missed without IV contrast enhancement.[4]

Initiation of Management

If an acute abdominopelvic injury is suspected, there are some principles of management that can be universally applied on the sideline (**Fig. 6**). The EAP should be promptly initiated. If safe to do so, keep the athlete in a supine position. The administration of IV fluids may be considered if the capability exists, especially if there are signs of shock (ie, hypotension and tachycardia/relative tachycardia). The definitive management of abdominopelvic trauma depends on the final diagnosis and severity of injury; specific considerations for the most commonly involved organs are detailed

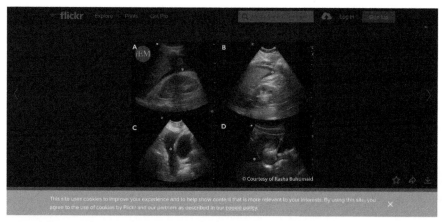

Fig. 5. Positive (abnormal) FAST examination (each image reflecting free fluid in the abdomen). (Courtesy of Dr. Rasha Buhumaid, MBBS, FACEP, ARDMS.)

below. As noted, there is a wide variety of therapies to consider depending on the diagnosis and severity of injury. For instance, a blood transfusion may be indicated in the setting of hemorrhagic shock, whereas IV antibiotics are indicated for intestinal perforation. In other instances, an interventional radiology procedure may be indicated for a liver laceration, whereas surgery may be indicated for a bladder rupture.

SPECIFIC DIAGNOSIS CONSIDERATIONS
Spleen

Evaluation
The spleen is the most commonly injured intra-abdominal organ in sport.[1,8] Mechanisms of injury may include direct trauma to the abdomen, a sudden deceleration impact (eg, an abrupt tackle in football), and/or displaced rib fractures causing a splenic laceration. It is also imperative to consider concomitant abdominal injuries in the setting of thorax trauma. In addition to trauma, a unique characteristic of the spleen is that infectious mononucleosis can cause spontaneous splenic rupture. Therefore, acute intrabdominal pathology should remain in the differential diagnosis in those with signs and symptoms of infectious mononucleosis with abdominal pain. A subsequent emergency department evaluation is likely to include laboratory testing including serial hemoglobin and hematocrit values as well as coagulation studies (ie, prothrombin time [PT]/international normalized ratio [INR], and partial thromboplastin time [PTT]) and type and crossmatch of blood, if needed. Imaging may include US and/or CT imaging[1,8,13] (**Fig. 7**).

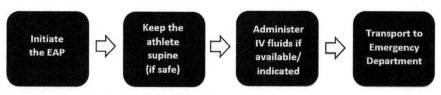

Fig. 6. Initiation of sideline management for abdominopelvic injuries.

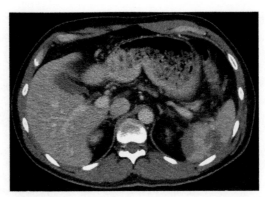

Fig. 7. Splenic rupture on CT. (CT Spleen Rupture, by Hellerhoff. https://commons. wikimedia.org/wiki/File:CT_Spleen_Rupture.jpg.)

Treatment

At minimum, patients with splenic lacerations are typically admitted to the hospital for observation including serial abdominal examinations, vital sign monitoring, and trending of hemoglobin and hematocrit values to evaluate for progression of the injury. Observation should occur in a facility with the capability of providing prompt reimaging and/or intervention (eg, by interventional radiology and/or general surgery) should the clinical status change (eg, increased pain, development of hypotension, and/or tachycardia). Nonoperative management is generally the course in hemodynamically stable patients regardless of injury grade. Embolization procedures serve as an adjunctive intervention as needed (eg, persistent bleeding in a hemodynamically stable patient). Hemodynamically unstable patients are likely to necessitate surgical intervention (eg, splenectomy).[1,8,13]

Outcome/return-to-play

No consensus guidelines exist for return-to-play following a splenic laceration. Generally, the timeline depends on the severity of injury. Return-to-play progression is appropriate once an appropriate time for healing has passed based on the initial grade of injury (**Table 1**), the associated pain has revolved, and any associated procedural wounds have healed.[1,13] In addition, return-to-baseline cardiopulmonary fitness should be completed before full participation.

Using mean time to healing data reduces the need for repeat US or CT imaging. Owing to the associated radiation exposure, repeat CT imaging is not recommended unless clinically indicated (eg, a change in patient status such as increased pain, development of hypotension, and/or tachycardia). Although return-to-play timelines should be individualized, general recommendations range from 6 weeks to 6 months for full return-to-play depending on the severity of injury. Non-consensus general recommendations for low-grade injuries (ie, grade I/II) include being restricted from all activity for 2 weeks with a return to full activity estimated at approximately 6 weeks for grade I injuries and 8 to 12 weeks for grade II injuries. High-grade injury (ie, grade III/IV) recommendations include performing activities of daily living only for 3 weeks with most recommendations suggesting a minimum of 3 months before a return to full activity.[1] There have been instances of high-level athletes choosing splenectomy or serial CT imaging in attempt to decrease the time to return-to-play; however, the risks and benefits of such management need to be thoroughly discussed before implementation.[1,8,13]

Table 1 Mean healing time for splenic lacerations	
Severity of Injury	Healing Time (wk)
Grade I	3.1
Grade II	8.2
Grade III	12.1
Grade IV	20.7

Data from Juyia RF, Kerr HA. Return to play after liver and spleen trauma. *Sports Health.* 2014 May; 6(3):239-45.

If splenectomy is necessary for management, it is important to remember that vaccinations certain for encapsulated organisms (ie, pneumococcal, meningococcal, and *Haemophilus influenzae*) are indicated.[1,8] In addition, it is recommended to follow the consensus guidelines for return-to-play in athletes with infectious mononucleosis secondary to an increased risk of splenic rupture.[1]

LIVER
Evaluation

Injury to the liver typically occurs secondary to a direct trauma to the RUQ and/or the lower right thorax. Deceleration injuries may also cause liver injuries.[1] If a liver injury is suspected, the emergent workup is likely to include laboratory analysis including hemoglobin and hematocrit values, liver function tests (eg, total bilirubin, alanine transaminase, aspartate transferase, and alkaline phosphatase), PT/INR, PTT, type and crossmatch of blood, and imaging including US and/or CT. Liver hematomas and lacerations are radiographically graded on a scale from I to VI, with VI being the most severe.[1,14,15]

Treatment

Management of liver hematomas and lacerations is similar to that of splenic injuries as detailed above. Ultimately, management depends on the patient's hemodynamic status with understanding that higher grade injuries (ie, IV–VI) have an increased likelihood of needing an interventional procedure such as embolization of a bleeding vessel or operative management. Patients with liver lacerations and/or hematomas are typically admitted to the hospital for observation including serial abdominal examinations, vital sign monitoring, and trending of hemoglobin, and hematocrit values. Observation should be performed in a facility with the capability of providing prompt reimaging and/or interventions should clinical status change (eg, increased pain, development of hypotension, and/or tachycardia).[1]

Outcome/Return-to-Play

For liver lacerations and hematomas, no consensus guidelines exist regarding return-to-play. However, normalization of liver enzymes and an appropriate time from injury for healing of the injury are necessary before returning to sport. In the past, time to healing was sometimes determined by repeat CT imaging.[4] However, serial CT scans are no longer considered the standard of care and are only indicated if clinical status changes.[4,14,15] Serial CT has been described in select cases of high-level athletes to facilitate a quicker return-to-play through evidence of radiographic healing with appropriate counseling of the risks of repeat CT imaging, including radiation exposure.[1]

Most of the liver lacerations, regardless of injury severity, heal within 4 months.[1,14,15] General recommendations include resuming progression toward normal activity approximately 3 to 4 months following the injury. Some low-grade injuries may result in a swifter return to activity, whereas high-grade injuries may necessitate up to 6 months before return-to-play. The final time to return-to-play necessitates an individualized plan in conjunction with clearance from any consultants (eg, general surgery). Liver enzymes should be normalized, and baseline cardiopulmonary fitness should be achieved.[1]

KIDNEY
Evaluation

Blunt renal trauma may occur in sport via a direct blow to the abdomen, back, and/or flank. In addition, high-velocity injuries (eg, a cycling crash, a ski jumping fall) can precipitate such an injury. In addition to abdominal or flank tenderness on examination, the presence of gross hematuria is a red flag for renal injury and should prompt emergent further evaluation.[6,16] Laboratory analysis in the emergent setting is likely to include hemoglobin and hematocrit values, PT/INR, PTT, type and crossmatch of blood, electrolyte testing (especially the creatinine level), and urinalysis.[6] Imaging including a CT with IV contrast (**Fig. 8**) is again the standard. The FAST examination may be used in a hemodynamically unstable patient to aid in determining if emergent surgical exploration is warranted.[6,16]

Treatment

Kidney injuries are also radiographically graded from I to V, with V being the most severe. Most of the sports-related renal injuries are low-grade (I–II). Most kidney injuries can be managed nonoperatively in hemodynamically stable patients. If the patient is hemodynamically unstable, an interventional radiology or surgical procedure may be indicated. Generally, all grades of kidney injuries are admitted to the hospital for monitoring of laboratory values and vital signs, symptom control, serial examinations,

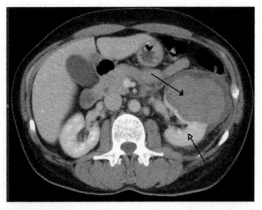

Fig. 8. Renal hematoma on CT (*open arrow*: renal parenchyma; *closed arrow*: renal hematoma). (Kidneyhematoma, by James Heilman, MD. https://commons.wikimedia.org/wiki/File:Kidneyhematoma.png.)

and reimaging if clinical status changes (ie, worsening pain, development of hypotension, and/or tachycardia).[6,16,17] Consideration for discharge from the emergency department may be an option for isolated low-grade injuries in the appropriate setting, including close follow-up and ability to return to the emergency department for any new or worsening symptoms.

Outcome/Return-to-Play

Renal injury return-to-play necessitates resolution of pain, healing of any procedural wound if present, resolution of hematuria (including microscopic hematuria), and a return-to-baseline cardiovascular fitness. Microscopic hematuria (ie, only seen on laboratory testing) may persist for approximately 4 to 6 weeks. Time to return-to-play is variable, but most of the sports-related renal injuries heal between 2 and 8 weeks with higher grade injuries requiring more healing time. The highest grade (V) kidney injuries may take substantially longer for return-to-play to contact sports.[6,16]

SMALL AND LARGE INTESTINES
Evaluation

Hollow viscus injuries of the abdomen (eg, traumatic bowel perforation) are fortunately rare in sport. Literature related to intestinal injuries in sport is primarily case reports related to contact sports resulting in direct trauma to the abdomen. The key point for hollow viscus injury is that a high index of suspicion should be maintained since the diagnosis is often delayed. Such a delay can lead to an increased risk of abdominal abscess and/or sepsis. The initial presentation may appear relatively benign with worsening symptoms more than the following several hours to days as peritonitis develops.[10,18] Fever, worsening pain, and increasing abdominal tenderness to palpation are concerning and should prompt emergent evaluation. The emergency department evaluation may include a laboratory analysis including but not limited to a complete blood count with differential, a complete metabolic panel, and a lactic acid if there is concern for sepsis. Subsequent imaging including a CT of the abdomen with IV contrast may be pursued (**Fig. 9**). As discussed above, abdominal plain films are of limited utility.

Treatment

Management depends on the severity of injury and systemic symptoms. Early recognition of the injury is imperative to decrease the likelihood of complications from intra-abdominal infection (eg, peritonitis, abscess). In the context of a delayed presentation, signs of sepsis necessitate IV fluid resuscitation and IV antibiotics. Hollow viscus injures (eg, a traumatic jejunal perforation) are highly likely to require a surgical intervention.[10] Intra-abdominal abscesses may develop, particularly later in an athlete's course, requiring further interventions including long-term antibiotics and/or drainage of the abscess.

Outcome/Return-to-Play

Hollow viscus injuries have high likelihood of necessitating a surgical intervention. The return-to-play timeline depends on the treating surgeon and time to wound healing. Generally, some progression is expected by 6 weeks after a surgical intervention. Confirmed intra-abdominal infection can lead to prolonged recovery secondary to an increased risk of complications (eg, intra-abdominal abscess) and likely need for long-term antibiotic therapy.[10]

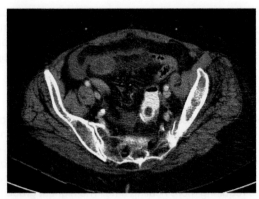

Fig. 9. Intestinal perforation on CT. (Galleinsteinperforation mit Duendarmnekrose - CT, by Hellerhoff. https://commons.wikimedia.org/wiki/File:Galleinsteinperforation_mit_Duendar mnekrose_-_CT_-_axial_-_012.jpg.)

PANCREAS
Evaluation

Pancreatic injury in sport is rarely reported in the literature. However, if present, a traumatic pancreatic injury has high morbidity and mortality, especially in the setting of delays in diagnosis greater than 24 hours, and thus needs to be included in the differential diagnosis of abdominopelvic trauma.[7] The mechanism of traumatic pancreatic injury is typically secondary to compression of the pancreas between the spine via an anteriorly applied high impact force to the abdomen.[7] The patient may present with epigastric and/or flank pain with tenderness to palpation on physical examination. A historical feature that should increase one's suspicion for pancreatic injury is pain that decreases more than the first 2 hours after injury and then increases again more than the next 6 to 8 hours. Laboratory analysis will likely include a complete blood count, a comprehensive metabolic panel, an amylase, and a lipase. A CT of the abdomen with IV contrast is typically secured to evaluate for potential pancreatic injury with transabdominal US serving as a potential imaging adjunct. If high clinical suspicion remains for pancreatic injury in the setting of a negative CT and/or US, a magnetic resonance cholangiopancreatography or endoscopic retrograde cholangiopancreatography may be obtained to further evaluate the pancreatic duct.[7,19]

Treatment

Patients with traumatic pancreatic injuries are typically admitted to the hospital. Management depends on the severity of injury, with higher grade injuries being associated with pancreatic duct injury. Management of low-grade injuries may consist of complete or partial bowel rest, IV hydration, and pain control. Higher grade injuries involving the pancreatic duct are likely to necessitate an intervention, such as pancreatic duct stenting and/or a surgical intervention.[7,19]

Outcome/Return-to-Play

There are no consensus guidelines regarding return-to-play following a traumatic pancreatic injury.[7,19] Symptoms of the injury should be resolved and any procedural wounds healed (if applicable) before consideration of return-to-sport. The athlete should have return of baseline cardiovascular fitness before full participation.[7]

RECTUS SHEATH HEMATOMA
Evaluation

Rectus sheath hematomas in sport are most often the result of direct trauma. The etiology of the hematoma is typically ruptured of an epigastric vein or artery. Presentation commonly includes focal pain and tenderness to palpation at the site of the hematoma. A visible or palpable abdominal mass may be present. The mass may continue to expand if active bleeding is present. The associated laboratory evaluation includes hemoglobin and hematocrit values, PT/INR, PTT, and often a CT of the abdomen with IV contrast (**Fig. 10**), which is the most sensitive (100%) imaging modality for rectus sheath hematoma.[20]

Treatment

Management depends on the hemodynamic status of the patient as well as the size of the hematoma. Hemodynamic instability and/or a persistently enlarging hematoma may necessitate IV fluids, blood transfusion, and/or an interventional radiology procedure (eg, arterial embolization). In a hemodynamically stable patient without a persistently enlarging hematoma, rest and observation may be the only indicated interventions.[21] Large hematomas greater than 7 cm in size and hematomas with active extravasation outside of the muscle, including hematomas that compromise overlying skin perfusion, may necessitate a surgical evacuation.[20,21]

Outcome/Return-to-Play

Return-to-play progression is appropriate once the associated pain resolves and procedural wounds have healed, if pertinent. As with all abdominopelvic injuries, a return-to-baseline cardiopulmonary fitness before full participation is necessary.

BLADDER RUPTURE
Evaluation

Traumatic bladder rupture in sport, while rare, is important to keep in the differential diagnosis for blunt abdominal trauma. Bladder injuries are often associated with other concomitant injuries, especially in the setting of pelvic fractures. Children and adolescents are at higher risk for isolated bladder rupture than adults due to the urinary bladder in children and adolescents being less protected by the developing bony

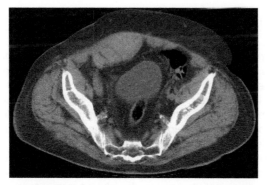

Fig. 10. Rectus sheath hematoma on CT. (Palatucci V, Lombardi G, Lombardi L, Giglio F, Giordano F, Lombardi D. Spontaneous muscle haematomas: management of 10 cases. Transl Med UniSa. 2014 Apr 8;10:13-7. PMID: 25147761; PMCID: PMC4140424.)

pelvis. In addition, having a full bladder at the time of injury also increases risk of isolated bladder rupture as the dome of a full bladder may not be well protected by the pelvic bones.[22,23] Signs and symptoms that should raise clinical suspicion for bladder injuries may include hematuria, gross blood at the urethral meatus, suprapubic tenderness, peritonitis, inability to void urine, and presence of a pelvic fracture.[22–24]

Owing to bladder rupture often being associated with other injuries, including pelvic fractures, it is common for multiple imaging modalities to be used during the emergency department evaluation. In a hemodynamically unstable patient, the FAST examination may be used to aid in determining the need for emergent exploratory laparotomy. In hemodynamically stable patients, plain radiographs of the pelvis and/or a CT with IV contrast may be used to evaluate for associated injuries. Specific to bladder injury, CT, or plain film cystography (depending on the facilities available resources) is recommended to evaluate for bladder injury if gross hematuria is present.[24]

Treatment

Management of bladder rupture is typically managed surgically. However, there is some debate as to whether all bladder ruptures necessitate surgical intervention depending on the precise location of the injury. If an intraperitoneal bladder rupture is diagnosed, surgical management is indicated.[24] Extraperitoneal bladder rupture management is more controversial and based on low-quality evidence. Extraperitoneal bladder ruptures that are classified as simple (ie, a single, full-thickness tear in the bladder wall resulting in spillage of urine into the extraperitoneal space) may potentially be managed nonoperatively, whereas extraperitoneal bladder ruptures classified as complex are managed operatively.[24]

Outcome/Return-to-Play

There are no standardized return-to-play guidelines following a bladder rupture. Therefore, a multidisciplinary approach to returning an athlete to sport should be undertaken. The surgical team should ensure that the injury and any associated wounds from the injury or repair of the injury have healed. The team physician and athletic training staff should ensure that any postsurgical restrictions are followed and develop a return-to-activity progression ensuring return-to-baseline cardiopulmonary fitness and strength are achieved.

TESTICULAR TRAUMA (TORSION/RUPTURE)
Evaluation

Blunt trauma to the scrotum can cause surgical emergencies, including testicular rupture as well as testicular torsion. After scrotal trauma, patients are likely to report immediate and severe pain.[25] Clinical evaluation may be difficult due to pain and swelling.[26] Associated nausea and vomiting may be present.[25] Additional history and physical examination in the setting of testicle rupture may include abnormal testicular contour and/or position on palpation, ecchymosis of the scrotum, and persistent pain.[25,26] Testicular torsion is the lack of blood flow to the testis secondary to the twisting of the spermatic cord and contents, including the testicular artery.[27,28] In testicular torsion, along with pain and possible nausea and/or vomiting, classic physical examination findings include a reduced or absent cremasteric reflex, a high-riding testicle, and/or abnormal position (ie, horizontally shifting) of the testicle.[27,28] Scrotal swelling and/or erythema may be present.

Emergent US, including color Doppler, is the imaging modality of choice for blunt testicular injuries.[25–28] If the US examination is inconclusive, but clinical suspicion remains high for a testicular rupture, MRI is recommended.[25] A color Doppler US revealing the lack of blood flow to the testis is 98% to 100% sensitive for the diagnosis of testicular torsion.[27,28] It should be noted that if the history and physical examination are concerning for testicular torsion, surgical consultation should not be delayed for the purpose of obtaining an imaging study.[28]

Treatment

For testicular rupture, early surgical exploration and repair are the recommended treatment strategy.[25,26] In the setting of testicular torsion, the goal is prompt restoration of blood flow to the testis. An attempt at manual detorsion of the testicle (ie, the open book maneuver of holding the testicle with the right thumb and forefinger followed by rotating the testicle clockwise 180° vs the opposite rotation in some cases) is immediately indicated at the bedside as long as it does not delay surgical intervention. Administration of an analgesic medication is recommended before attempting manual detorsion. Even if symptoms improve with manual detorsion, emergent surgical exploration is still indicated.[27,28]

Outcome/Return-to-Play

There are no consensus guidelines regarding return-to-play following a testicular rupture or testicular torsion. Symptoms including pain should be resolved, and any wounds from the injury or surgical interventions should be healed before return-to-play. If an orchiectomy is necessary the athlete should be counseled on wearing appropriate protective equipment (ie, athletic cup) to aid in preserving the remaining testicle should another injury occur to the area. In the setting of testicular rupture, follow-up regarding fertility considerations, including monitoring for antisperm antibody and testosterone levels, should be considered.[25]

SUMMARY

Abdominopelvic injuries can be challenging on the sideline due to varying presentations, the potential for life-threatening pathology, and limited diagnostic and therapeutic modalities available. The sideline physician should focus on the early identification of the signs and symptoms necessitating further workup, timely transportation for further evaluation and management, and implementation of stabilizing procedures using the tools available on the sideline.

There are no consensus guidelines for return-to-play from traumatic abdominopelvic injury. Consequently, return-to-play decisions need to be individualized based on the patient's injury, interventions implemented, and recovery course. Applying average healing times based on the grade of injury for splenic and liver lacerations may aid in these decisions.[1] Pathologies necessitating surgical interventions require enough time for wound healing and resolution of the original injury. Athletes should be symptom-free and return to their baseline fitness level before returning to full participation.

CLINICS CARE POINTS

- Maintain a high index of suspicion for intestinal rupture/perforation as a delay in diagnosis can result in the development of abscess and/or sepsis.

> • Reimaging injuries (eg, splenic lacerations), particularly with computed tomography, to evaluate for healing is not routinely recommended.

DISCLOSURE

The authors have nothing to disclose.

REFERENCES

1. Juyia RF, Kerr HA. Return to play after liver and spleen trauma. Sports Health 2014;6(3):239–45.
2. Chen A, Archbold C, Hutchinson M, et al. Sideline management of nonmusculoskeletal injuries by the orthopaedic team physician. JAAOS 2019;27(4):e146–55.
3. Johnson BK, Comstock RD. Epidemiology of chest, rib, thoracic spine, and abdomen injuries among United States high school athletes, 2005/06 to 2013/14. Clin J Sport Med 2017;27(4):388–93.
4. Walter KD. Radiographic Evaluation of the patient with sport-related abdominal trauma. Curr Sports Med Rep 2007;6(2):115–9.
5. Weinstein S, Khodaee M, VanBaak K. Common skiing and snowboarding injuries. Curr Sports Med Rep 2019;18(11):394–400.
6. Bernard JJ. Renal trauma. Curr Sports Med Rep 2009;8(2):98–103.
7. Echlin PS, Klein WB. Pancreatic injury in the athlete. Curr Sports Med Rep 2005; 4(2):96–101.
8. Gannon EH, Howard T. Splenic injuries in athletes. Curr Sports Med Rep 2010; 9(2):111–4.
9. Rahbour G, Ullah MR, Yassin N, et al. Cullen's sign - case report with a review of the literature. Int J Surg Case Rep 2012;3(5):143–6.
10. Phillips S, Seidenberg P, Onks C, et al. Sport-related jejunal rupture. Curr Sports Med Rep 2019;18(3):68–71.
11. Richards J, McGahan J. Focused Assessment with Sonography in Trauma (FAST) in 2017: What Radiologists Can Learn. Radiology 2017;283(1):30–48.
12. Hahn M, Ray J, Hall M, et al. Ultrasound in trauma and other acute conditions in sports, part I. Curr Sports Med Rep 2020;19(11):486–94.
13. Terrell TR, Lundquist B. Management of splenic rupture and return-to-play decisions in a college football player. Clin J Sport Med 2002;12(6):400–2.
14. Coccolini F, Catena F, Moore EE, et al. WSES classification and guidelines for liver trauma. World J Emerg Surg 2016;11(50).
15. Coccolini F, Coimbra R, Ordonez C, et al. WSES expert panel. Liver trauma: WSES 2020 guidelines. World J Emerg Surg 2020;15(1):24.
16. Freeman CM, Kelly ME, Nason GJ, et al. Renal trauma: the rugby factor. Current Urology 2015;8(3):133–7.
17. Erlich T, Kitrey ND. Renal trauma: the current best practice. Ther Adv Urol 2018; 10(10):295–303.
18. Browne GJ, Noaman F, Lam LT, et al. The nature and characteristics of abdominal injuries sustained during children's sports. Pediatr Emerg Care 2010;26(1):30–5.
19. Cully M, Perry J, Titus M. An unlikely cause of a blunt pancreatic injury. Pediatr Emerg Care 2019;35(12):e238–40.
20. Hatjipetrou A, Anyfantakis D, Kastanakis M. Rectus sheath hematoma: a review of the literature. Int J Surg 2015;13:267–71.

21. Liao ED, Puckett Y. A Proposed Algorithm on the Modern Management of Rectus Sheath Hematoma: A Literature Review. Cureus 2021;13(11):e20008.

22. Nicola R, Menias CO, Mellnick V, et al. Sports-related genitourinary trauma in the male athlete. Emerg Radiol 2015;22:157–68.

23. Phillips B, Holzmer S, Turco L, et al. Trauma to the bladder and ureter: a review of diagnosis, management, and prognosis. Eur J Trauma Emerg Surg 2017;43: 763–73.

24. Yeung LL, McDonald AA, Como JJ, et al. Management of blunt force bladder injuries: A practice management guideline from the Eastern Association for the Surgery of Trauma. *J. Trauma Acute Care Surg*. February 2019;86(2):326–36.

25. Wang Z, Yang JR, Huang YM, et al. Diagnosis and management of testicular rupture after blunt scrotal trauma: a literature review. Int Urol Nephrol 2016;48: 1967–76.

26. Essien F, Eagle Z, Tate J, et al. Testicular Rupture: The Other Nutcracker Syndrome. *Clin Med Insights* Case Rep 2022;15. 11795476211052416.

27. Manjunath AS, Hofer MD. Urologic Emergencies. Med Clin North Am 2018; 102(2):373–85.

28. Sharp VJ, Kieran K, Arlen AM. Testicular torsion: diagnosis, evaluation, and management. Am Fam Physician 2013;88(12):835–40.

General Medical Emergencies in Athletes

Jens T. Verhey, MD[a], Steven K. Poon, MD, CAQSM[b],*

KEYWORDS

- Sports medicine • Asthma • Sudden cardiac arrest • Emergency action plan

KEY POINTS

- The key element of on-field emergency management in sports is a well-prepared team and primary prevention of medical emergencies.
- All emergency action plans should be reviewed on an annual basis to reflect the needs of individual athletes with any complex medical problems and the skills of the physician.
- Immediate, local, and regional medical resources should be factored as part of primary prevention planning or screening.

INTRODUCTION

This article focuses on the management of the most common on-field medical emergencies. As with any discipline in medicine, a well-defined plan and systematic approach is the cornerstone of quality health care delivery. In addition, team-based collaboration is necessary for the safety of the athlete and the success of the treatment plan. This is especially true when care is delivered on the field, as the environment can be hectic and fraught with distraction. In this section, the principles of emergency preparedness will be described in detail with particular focus on the most encountered medical conditions affecting athletes during practice and competition.

EMERGENCY PREPAREDNESS AND DEVELOPING AN ACTION PLAN

Athletic sideline coverage is simultaneously exciting and highly demanding for the sports medicine physician and health care team. Although most on-field injuries are low acuity, it is essential to have a well-organized protocol for the rare life- or limb-threatening emergency. This protocol is best summarized by the emergency action plan (EAP), which details the roles and responsibilities of each member of the care team should an emergent medical event occur. EAPs allow for timely, multidisciplinary

[a] Orthopaedic Surgery Residency, Department of Orthopaedic Surgery, Mayo Clinic Arizona, Phoenix, AZ, USA; [b] Sports Medicine Section, Department of Orthopaedic Surgery, Mayo Clinic Arizona, Phoenix, AZ, USA
* Corresponding author.
E-mail address: poon.steven@mayo.edu

Clin Sports Med 42 (2023) 427–440
https://doi.org/10.1016/j.csm.2023.02.007
0278-5919/23/© 2023 Elsevier Inc. All rights reserved.

care to be delivered in the most effective manner possible, thus ensuring that the athlete has the best outcome possible.

EAPs are written with several components in mind including logistical factors, personnel, equipment, information about the sporting venue, communication procedures, transportation modalities, and quickest access to an emergency care facility.[1] The written documentation of the EAP should include key personnel at the sporting venue with their roles, respective contact information, office location, location during practice and competition times, and alternative contacts should they not be available at the time of injury. If certain key personnel are not present at the time of the game, such as the athletic trainer and team physician, then the competition cannot ensue. Resuscitation equipment, its location, and prerequisite training for use should be specified next. Equipment should be listed with respect to the possible acuity of its use. Therefore, cardiopulmonary resuscitation devices, including a defibrillator, bag-mask airway, and medications should be listed first, followed by equipment related to hemorrhage control (pelvic binder and tourniquets). In addition, a clear map of the facility with prespecified exit routes should be included along with detailed instructions for exit procedures. Ideally, multiple exit routes should exist if one route is inaccessible or obstructed. Transportation modalities should be listed, including ambulance presence, with threshold criteria for activating emergency response transportation beyond car transit to health care services. Again, the EAP should clearly define that competition cannot be initiated if the necessary transportation modalities are not present on-site. Finally, nearby health care facilities, including a Level I Trauma Center, should be clearly designated within the EAP. Alongside the facility listing should be threshold criteria to transfer a patient to each of these facilities with recommended route of transportation.

THE PRIMARY SURVEY

The main objective of the primary survey is rapid identification and treatment of life-threatening injuries. Consequently, the primary survey should be conducted in a timely fashion by the most senior clinician present on the field in concert with various support staff. Leveraging the skills of the entire team is essential to delivering optimal care within the first hour of a trauma, the organization of which depends on the physician. In the athletic setting, the most common causes leading to morbidity and mortality are airway obstruction, hemorrhage, head injury, and cardiopulmonary arrest,[2] all of which are assessed with the primary survey. Examining the athlete for signs of airway obstruction, internal or external hemorrhage, respiratory depression or arrest, pneumothorax, focal neurologic compromise, and increased intracranial pressure is the hallmarks of a thorough primary survey. A complete history and physical examination should be reserved for the secondary survey so as not to delay critical, life-saving resuscitation processes.

At the time of the primary survey, all team members should ensure that they are wearing the appropriate personal protective equipment, such as masks, gloves, eyewear, and gowns. The patient should be positioned to allow for full assessment of injuries and to facilitate treatment with efficiency of movement. Roles and responsibilities should be clearly defined by the leader briefly as the resuscitation process begins. These roles consist of (1) a team leader who facilitates the management plan, (2) management of the airway, ventilation, and cervical spine stabilization, (3) management of circulation, chest compressions, and exposure of the thorax and abdomen, (4) control of appropriate resuscitation equipment and medications, including the defibrillator, (5) call for emergency services, and (6) communications with family members, teammates, and other surrounding observers. Critical equipment should be readily available as the team reaches the injured athlete, including a stethoscope for cardio-pulmonary examination, a pulse oximeter to assess oxygenation, and supplies to secure the airway, including a bag-mask device and oropharyngeal airway.

The first step of the primary survey is safely obtaining control of the airway and cervical spine. Establishing a patent airway should be completed in tandem with cervical spine stabilization, especially if the witnessed injury mechanism involved head or spine trauma. The airway is assumed to be patent if the patient can respond coherently. However, attention should be made to continually reassess the airway should an obstruction develop. The cervical spine is stabilized by ensuring that the face, neck, and body remain in the same coronal plane when shifting position. This process may require two individuals, particularly if a helmet or other equipment needs to be removed. One team member should ensure proper neck alignment, whereas another team member carefully removes the helmet or other equipment impeding assessment of the airway. As helmets have unique designs and release mechanisms, the individual responsible for its removal should ideally be familiar with the equipment. Each team member should be familiar with the fitting and sizing of a cervical collar, which should be placed at this juncture to assist with stabilization. If the patient is unresponsive, performing a chin lift or jaw thrust after ensuring cervical spine stability is essential to determine whether airway obstruction is present. The jaw thrust maneuver is performed by placing fingertips at the angle of the mandible, the thumbs under the chin, and lifting anteriorly. A foreign body should be promptly removed at this time if identified. Even if an obstruction is not visualized, the jaw thrust maneuver allows for expansion of the airway and improved gas exchange whether the patient is breathing spontaneously or requires resuscitation. Supplemental oxygen can be administered to the patient; it should be assumed that no contraindication to the administration of oxygen is present in the primary survey phase. Finally, facial trauma should also be assessed at this time.

Ensuring a patent airway is critical; however, the physician must also determine whether the athlete is adequately ventilating and oxygenating. Adequate exposure of the chest and abdomen is essential to determine whether tracheal deviation, chest wounds, paradoxic chest movement, and flail chest are present at the time of injury. Lung sounds should be auscultated to determine symmetric and spontaneous ventilation. Passive ventilation with bag-mask device or rescue breaths should be administered if the patient is not spontaneously respirating. Decreased lung sounds paired with deviated trachea may be indicative of pneumothorax or hemothorax. If the athlete has clinical signs of pneumothorax in the setting of hemodynamic compromise, tension pneumothorax should be suspected and promptly treated with needle decompression and thoracotomy tube placement. Finally, any chest wounds should be bandaged to prevent propagation of atmospheric air entry into the chest which may spur on or worsen pneumothorax.

Blood circulation and hemorrhage control are turned to next. The physician should determine whether the patient is suffering from hemodynamic compromise and shock. In the athletic and trauma setting, hypovolemic shock secondary to hemorrhage is the most common reason for hemodynamic compromise and any readily apparent external bleeding should be controlled with direct pressure and/or tourniquets to the extremities. If there is concern for abdominopelvic trauma and intrapelvic hemorrhage, a pelvic binder or sheet should be applied to tamponade blood loss. The patient's level of responsiveness (or lack thereof) correlates with the shock state and is determined by whether a patient is alert, responsive to verbal stimuli, responsive to painful stimuli, or altogether unresponsive.[3] In addition, pale skin, increased capillary refill time, and weak pulses in the carotids and femoral arteries are all signs concerning for significant hypovolemia. A patient suffering from hemorrhage will maintain their baseline blood pressure until losing approximately 30% of their total blood volume, as the body compensates with peripheral vasoconstriction. Therefore, even mild hypotension is an indicator of large volume blood loss.

Although the level of responsiveness has already been established, further neurologic evaluation is necessary to determine the extent of the patient's disability. The Glasgow Coma Scale (GCS) is the most critical portion of the primary survey with motor, verbal, and eye responsiveness components. A maximum GCS score of 15 indicates full consciousness, whereas a score below 3 indicates a deep coma. In addition, a score below 8 signifies that a patient is unable to protect their own airway necessitating a definitive airway. In the absence of a known head trauma, a reduced GCS score may be a sign of cerebral hypoxia or hypoperfusion.

The final portion of the primary survey relates to exposure and environmental control. Adequate exposure of the patient is essential for a complete evaluation of their injuries. Failure to obtain necessary exposure may result in untreated injuries which lead to significant morbidity and mortality for the patient. Therefore, the treating physician and care team should never assume that an uncovered area of the body is injury free. By the same token, ensuring adequate exposure also means ensuring privacy for the patient. Because the field or arena is limited with regard to privacy and confidentiality, it is the responsibility of the care team to protect the patient from observers and the patient should be transferred to the medical tent or secure locker room whenever it is safe to do so. Furthermore, the care team should make every effort that the patient remains normothermic, especially as they may not be able to autoregulate their temperature in the trauma setting.

THE SECONDARY SURVEY

After the care team has completed a primary survey and the patient is adequately stabilized, a secondary survey can be completed with the goal of obtaining a detailed history, complete physical examination, and full systems review. It is important to ensure that all life- and limb-threatening conditions have been addressed and vital signs have normalized. If the patients were to have a clinical decline during the secondary survey process, then the primary survey must be promptly reinitiated. A detailed history should be obtained as part of the secondary survey with a focus on age and sex of the patient, mechanism of injury, signs and symptoms, last oral intake, previous medical history, and medications. When discussing the mechanism of injury, specific focus on blunt versus penetrating trauma is highly useful to determine next workup and treatment steps.

A thorough secondary survey physical examination begins with the head and neck. The scalp should be examined for hematoma, depression fracture, or laceration with careful palpation. In addition, the facial bony margins of the maxilla, nose, orbits, and mandible should be palpated. The ears should be evaluated for ecchymosis or hemotympanum, which may be a sign of basilar skull fracture. Pupillary response and ocular mobility should be performed to rule out entrapment. If signs concerning for basilar skull fracture or cerebrospinal fluid leak are present, the care team should refrain from placing a nasogastric tube. The neck should be examined without compromise of stability with chief concern for edema or pulsatile neck mass.

The chest wall should be palpated for tenderness and crepitus. The clavicles and sternum are common sites of fracture that require additional attention due to nearby neurovascular structures. Cardiopulmonary auscultation should be performed with attention to symmetric breath sounds and clear, non-muffled heart sounds. The abdomen should then be assessed for distention, ecchymosis, and focal pain. The perineum should be inspected for ecchymosis or laceration. However, digital rectal and vaginal examinations should be reserved for situations where there is high suspicion for pelvic injury and fracture indicated by point tenderness, instability, and step-offs along the pelvic ring. If blood is present at the urethral meatus, urethral injury should be anticipated and a retrograde urethrogram should be obtained before placing a Foley catheter.

The extremities should be assessed for fracture or joint dislocation by palpation along their entire length. Active and passive range of motion can be evaluated at this time along with a neurovascular examination. Findings of the neurovascular examination should be documented and tracked over time. Careful attention should be given to palpating each compartment in the extremity to rule out compartment syndrome. Tense compartments with pain out of proportion on examination require urgent decompression.

CONSTRUCTING A FIRST-AID KIT

As modern sports medicine has progressed, most equipment is available on site at various athletic facilities. However, a universal sports medicine kit or equipment bag should be in close reach for the physician at all athletic coverage events. An appropriately constructed sports medicine first-aid kit should include personal protective equipment, tools for airway management, cardiovascular assessment and resuscitation, wound care supplies, immobilization and splinting materials, tourniquet, sphygmomanometer, thermometer, glucometer, and emergency use medications. These general classes of instrumentation are directed at handling most medical emergencies in children and adults until emergency services arrive on scene.

DIABETES, HYPOGLYCEMIA, AND INSULIN SHOCK

As diabetes prevalence expands in the population, so does the number of athletes affected by diabetes. Diabetic athletes range extensively in age and skill level, from youth participants to professional and Olympic champions, and each presents a unique set of challenges to the physicians who care for them. With high metabolic demands in practice and competition, these athletes are at an elevated risk for hypoglycemic episodes, ketoacidosis, insulin shock, and secondary complications from diabetes-associated vasculopathies and neuropathies.

Approximately 90% of patients with diabetes are type 2 and are more frequently encountered than type 1.[4] Type 1 diabetes mellitus (T1DM) is typically early onset in youth, adolescence, or young adulthood but can initially present at any age due to the lack of insulin production. Type 2 diabetes mellitus (T2DM) is the result of insulin resistance coupled with reduced insulin secretion. The onset of T2DM occurs as a gradual progression due to various lifestyle factors, as hypertension, hyperglycemia, central adipose distribution, and dyslipidemia usually predate diagnosis by as much as 10 to 20 years. T2DM occurs in patients primarily with metabolic syndrome; however, there is a genetic predisposition to developing the condition. Although T2DM is less likely to affect the athletic population, special consideration must be given to athletes with increased body mass index, including baseball players, football lineman, and golfers. Athletes with T1DM require more frequent monitoring, as they are subject to ketosis.

Treatment plans are primarily guided by the type of diabetes and chosen sport. Factors such as intensity, duration, and aerobic versus anaerobic-type exercise are all variables to be considered in preparing for the diabetic athlete's care. It is well-established that aerobic exercise leads to hypoglycemia, whereas bursts of anaerobic exercise may elevate blood glucose levels.[5] On the individual level, the physician should encourage the athlete to monitor their performance at varying glycemic levels and the athlete should also be cognizant of their symptoms when approaching hypoglycemia. Likewise, the coaching and health care staff should be aware of signs of metabolic encephalopathy related to glucose level derangement, especially during head-to-head competition when other players may be at risk. Finally, careful attention must be applied to nutritional needs before, during, and after training for athletes with diabetes.

The demand of exercise requires a physiologic cascade of events driven by hormones and the sympathetic nervous system. Through the breakdown of glycogen in the muscle and liver, gluconeogenesis in the liver and kidneys, and beta oxidation of fatty acid stores, energy is freed to use for physical activity. Previously, exercise has been shown to increase insulin sensitivity primarily by facilitating glucose transport across the cell by membrane glucose transporter 4 (GLUT-4).[6] This modulation of the GLUT-4 receptor has a lasting effect after exercise, as a 45-minute session of moderately intense activity can increase insulin sensitivity for up to 48 hours. The diabetic athlete is at increased risk for hypoglycemia during exercise and for an extended period afterward. Controlling blood glucose levels is further complicated by variable absorption rates and dosing routes of exogenous insulin.

In concert with their athletic trainer and team physician, the athlete should have predefined blood glucose levels at which it is safe to practice and compete. When available, registered dietitians with expertise in sports populations also provide valuable benefit to the athlete care team. In addition, their nutritional and hydration needs should be modified based on a pre-exercise glucose level. Early and frequent blood glucose monitoring should occur at minimum 90 minutes before exercise, ideally with two to three measurements to ensure the athlete is aware of their glucose trend. If the pre-exercise level is determined to be range between 100 and 250 mg/dL, it is acceptable to begin exercise; however, most athletes should attempt to maintain blood glucose levels above 200 mg/dL. The athlete should supplement with carbohydrate-rich nutrition should they fall below this range. If the athlete falls above this range, they should instead focus on hydration with a noncarbohydrate-containing fluid to prevent dehydration. Serum glucose levels should be monitored every 30 minutes, and the nutrition and hydration plan should continuously be altered. Anaerobic and short-duration exercise has minimal effect on glucose levels, and the corresponding adjustment of insulin dosage is often unnecessary. Transient hyperglycemia may be induced by short bursts of activity due to catecholamine release. By contrast, endurance athletes may decrease long-acting insulin dosage in anticipation of exercise.

Hypoglycemia most often occurs during activity secondary to inadequate nutrition, low pre-exercise glucose levels, or excessive exogenous insulin. Importantly, insulin should not be injected into or near muscles active during exercise which can lead to increased absorption rate.[7] Longer duration of exercise in cold conditions demands higher calorie intake leading to the increased risk of hypoglycemia. In hot weather conditions, athletes may become hypoglycemic due to decreased appetite.

Most symptoms that athletes report are the result of increased adrenergic activity, including anxiety, diaphoresis, tremor, and irregular heartbeat. Symptoms of neuroglycopenia are most apparent to other observers; athletic trainers and physicians should be cognizant of fatigue, confusion, stupor, and slowed or uncoordinated speech as signs of hypoglycemia. Furthermore, younger athletes are more likely to experience seizures or loss of consciousness than adults when the brain has insufficient glucose supply.[8]

When an athlete becomes aware of symptoms or an observer suspects hypoglycemia, a simple carbohydrate source of 20 g in the form of a tablet or juice can resolve symptoms quickly and an initial supplementation should be given 15 minutes to take effect. A complex carbohydrate can be ingested before returning to play to prevent recurrence. Although the athlete may have an appetite for additional carbohydrate, care should be taken to avoid hyperglycemic rebound which would further delay return to game and place the athlete at risk for ketosis if dehydration is also present.[9]

Glucose levels should be checked frequently after exercise. Delayed post-exertional hypoglycemia can occur,[10] usually between 6 and 12 hours post-exercise, but can have onset up to 28 hours after activity.[11] When the hypoglycemic event occurs at nighttime or during sleep, athletes may be subject to insidious cardiac and neurologic complications. Consequently, athletes should be encouraged to replenish their nutrition stores in the hours following exercise, especially as insulin sensitivity rises after activity.[12] Adequate replenishment consists of 1.5 g of carbohydrate per kilogram body weight.[13]

Life-threatening hypoglycemia with altered mentation, significant lethargy, seizures, and loss of consciousness requires rapid intervention by athletic staff and the emergency medical team. A diabetic athlete who becomes unresponsive on the field is subject to hypoglycemia until proven otherwise. Because of aspiration risk, treatment with oral carbohydrates is not indicated. The intramuscular administration of glucagon is the first-choice treatment given its ease and rapidity, especially when trained medical providers are not present. Recovery after administration of glucagon usually leads to symptomatic resolution within 15 minutes but may be followed by significant nausea and emesis. When the athlete regains consciousness, they should be given carbohydrate supplementation, as the effects of glucagon are transient. If an athlete is on a sulfonylurea medication, a longer duration and quantity of carbohydrate supplementation may be required due to persistent insulin secretion stimulation by the medication class.

AIRWAY REACTIVITY AND ASTHMA

Epidemiologic studies have found that the prevalence of asthma is higher among athletes than the general population, with rates as high as 19.3% in regular exercisers.[14,15] Team medical staff and coaches should be acutely aware that even mild asthma can become an on-field emergency in the setting of exercise-induced bronchoconstriction. Athletes with a diagnosis of asthma should be well-documented as they are at higher risk for complication.

Asthma is a dynamic obstructive airway condition which is worsened by thermal changes and increased minute ventilation. During exercise, increased ventilation leads to cooling of the airway by vaporization and dehydration of the airway. Increasing osmolarity of the respiratory lining leads to the production and release of inflammatory mediators, including histamine, prostaglandins, and leukotrienes.[16] These mediators lead to hyperemia of the mucosa and bronchoconstriction impairing gas exchange. In addition, the respiratory system is subject to increased pollutant exposure as mouth breathing is a common practice during intense activity.[17,18] Swimmers and athletes participating in winter sports are more likely to suffer from reactive airway disease, with exposure cold, dry air, and chloramines, respectively.[19,20] Athletes are at a continued risk of post-exercise due to airway rewarming and continued release of inflammatory factors.

An asthma action plan is the cornerstone of treatment in both athletes and nonathletes to optimize respiratory function and minimize the risk of acute exacerbation. Education about asthma self-treatment is an important primary step to prevent acute worsening of symptoms. The health care team should ensure that athletes competing with asthma are under control before starting activity. Although short-acting β2-agonists (SABA) are the preferred treatment of mild, intermittent asthma, those athletes who become symptomatic greater than twice per week should be initiated on a daily inhaled low-dose glucocorticoid. A daily dosage of inhaled glucocorticoid is more effective than a SABA at directly counteracting the reactive airway response induced by exercise by reducing inflammatory mediators.[21] Leukotriene-receptor antagonists are a useful adjunctive therapy when an inhaled glucocorticoid is not sufficient as maintenance therapy.[22] However, caution should be used when initiating this medication as the United States Food and Drug Administration (FDA) issued a warning in 2020 about serious mental health side effects. When pre-exercise control is obtained, athletes should be counseled on the protective effects of a mild-to-moderate intensity warm-up in reducing the effects of bronchoconstriction during intense exercise.[23] This is thought to be due to a tachyphylactic mechanism in which prostaglandin release before exercise downregulates the bronchoconstriction response.[23]

For suspected acute exacerbations occurring on-field, the athlete should be removed from play immediately and assessed for clinical signs of airway compromise. This includes the use of accessory muscles to breathe, inability to speak, altered mental status, and inability to lie supine. Heightened concern should be present when the athlete presents with cyanosis or a fatiguing respiratory drive. The initial medical management consists of inhaled SABA every 20 minutes after removal from play with continuous monitoring of symptoms. If resources are available, additional therapy with oxygen supplementation, long-acting muscarinic antagonists, and systemic glucocorticoids is indicated for moderate-to-severe exacerbations. Oral prednisone or intramuscular (IM) methylprednisolone is preferred for on-field management. Ipratropium bromide is an effective inhaled muscarinic antagonist that should be administered with the SABA inhaler every 20 minutes. In patients who are unable to use inhaled treatments, either epinephrine IM or terbutaline given subcutaneously are reasonable alternatives that can be given every 20 minutes for three doses. Importantly, these medications should not be given together.

The decision to secure an airway before emergency services arrival is based on clinical judgment and requires the appropriate expertise available on-site. In the setting of decreased respiratory rate and unresponsiveness, an endotracheal airway should be obtained. The patient should be ventilated with low tidal volumes and low respiratory rates to avoid barotrauma.

The prevalence of asthma and exercise-induced bronchoconstriction is estimated at 70% among the athletic population. Emergent exacerbations are best avoided with preemptive control of the reactive airway with an asthma action plan.

SEIZURE DISORDER

As pharmacologic management of seizure disorders improves and stigmatization of epilepsy decreases, those with seizure disorders have become progressively more active in athletics. The most recent recommendation by the International League Against Epilepsy (ILAE) was released in 1997 indicating that patients with epilepsy should be encouraged to participate in all forms of athletic activity except for scuba diving and skydiving. Water sports, cycling, and activities involving heights, such as rock climbing, are safe with adequate seizure control (ILAE 1997). Indeed, regular participation in sporting activities has demonstrated positive physiologic and psychosocial benefits for those with epilepsy. Exercise can induce the production of endogenous seizure-inhibitory neurotransmitters gamma amino butyric acid and adenosine.

Multiple clinical studies have elucidated the benefits and safety of physical activity for patients with epilepsy. Furthermore, repetitive minor head trauma does not lead to increased frequency or severity of seizure activity.[24]

Noncontact aerobic activities, including running, hiking, and cycling, are particularly beneficial for those with epilepsy while minimizing the risk present in contact sports. Both the American Medical Association (AMA) and American Academy of Pediatrics (AAP) encourage participation without restriction, as seizures triggered by these activities are very rare. Contact sports, including football, soccer, and hockey, are also safe for participation. Even activities with repetitive blows to the head do not increase the risk of seizure activity, as karate and judo have been shown to have a protective effect.[24]

Although rare, seizure activity can occur on the field in both athletes with known epilepsy and those without a previous seizure disorder diagnosis. There are many mimickers of seizure and motor movements associated with a syncopal episode often resemble a myoclonic seizure event including sudden cardiac arrest in athletes. Thus, any unprovoked witnessed collapse with myoclonic movements in a sports setting should raise concern for serious cardiac event. In addition, seizure must be distinguished from psychogenic nonepileptic seizures and convulsive concussions. Underlying etiologies of seizure provocation must also be considered, including hypoglycemia and alcohol withdrawal.

On-field management of seizure first requires supportive care with direct attention to airway, breathing, and circulation. Every effort should be made to position the patient in the lateral decubitus position to prevent aspiration. An electrocardiogram (ECG) and oxygenation status should be promptly monitored. Finally, a blood glucose level should be assessed and a brief neurologic examination performed. Transfer of the patient off the playing field should not be attempted until seizure activity is under control.

A single generalized seizure with complete recovery does not necessitate pharmacologic management. However, when the athlete is in status epilepticus (two or more sequential seizures without full recovery or more than 30 minutes of continuous seizure activity), antiepileptic drug therapy should be initiated after airway, breathing, and circulation factors are assessed. In settings where an athlete with known history of epilepsy is monitored only by an athletic trainer or coach, an EAP and training should be developed for administration of benzodiazepine via sublingual, or more effectively, rectal route. Otherwise, lorazepam administered IV or IM every 2 minutes is the preferred initial treatment. Care should be taken to continuously assess airway and respiratory rate, as respiratory depression, hypotension, and sialorrhea are expected with benzodiazepine administration, particularly with repetitive dosing.

Many systemic complications can occur after prolonged seizure activity. Increased metabolic activity in the setting of decreased oxygenation can lead to lactic acidosis, hypercapnia, and hypoglycemia. The patient may be subject to hyperpyrexia, vomiting, and incontinence due to seizure interference with the autonomic system. Finally, devastating complications including acute renal failure secondary to rhabdomyolysis along with cardiac arrhythmia and respiratory failure are possible if status epilepticus is not managed promptly.

SUNBURN AND OTHER DERMATOLOGIC CONDITIONS

Ultraviolet-A (UVA) and ultraviolet-B (UVB) radiation play a role in acute sunburn; however, UVB rays are the primary etiology of DNA damage and inflammatory sequelae. UVB radiation damages DNA by causing formation of thymine–thymine cyclobutane dimers leading to a DNA repair response, apoptosis of cells, and release of inflammatory mediators such as prostaglandins, bradykinin, and reactive oxygen species.[25,26] On clinical evaluation, these inflammatory factors lead to the vasogenic edema, redness, and pain characteristic of a sunburn.

Signs of excessive sun exposure include erythema, pain, and blistering that are proportional to the intensity and duration of ultraviolet (UV) radiation. In the context of athletic activity, the athlete may have challenges with fatigue and ability to self-regulate temperature, impairing their ability to return to practice or competition. Severe sunburns can lead to additional systemic symptoms, including nausea and fevers even after the athlete is removed from exposure.

If the burn is mild without signs of full thickness burn (including blistering and edema), the athlete may return to play after application of sunscreen. Perspiration- and water-resistant formulas are preferred with sun protection factor (SPF) of at least 30 applied more than 30 minutes before exposure and every 90 minutes subsequently. UV-resistant clothing can be used in conjunction. For moderate and severe burns, the athlete should be removed from play and sun exposure to avoid further skin damage. The athlete should be encouraged to drink additional water, as fluid loss into the skin interstitium may occur due to the inflammatory response. Non-steroidal inflammatories can be used for anti-inflammatory effects, minimizing the production of prostaglandins and leukotrienes. Furthermore, topical creams such as aloe vera or corticosteroid can be helpful for symptomatic and anti-inflammatory effects, respectively. Intravenous fluid resuscitation may be required in cases of severe burn with signs of low effective arterial volume due to capillary fluid leak. In these cases, the Parkland formula is useful to calculate the appropriate resuscitation volume.

Importantly, sunburn must be distinguished from other etiologies, including systemic lupus erythematosus, dermatomyositis, infection, rosacea, stasis dermatitis, and photoallergic reactions. Erythema which does not resolve after sun exposure may require further workup for underlying disease, especially with accompanying symptoms.

HEAT EXHAUSTION AND HEATSTROKE

Heat-related injury can be associated with rapid deterioration and death when not assessed and treated appropriately. Although common sense would indicate that heat injury primarily affects athletes practicing and competing in hot-humid climates with large amounts of protective gear, heat exhaustion and heatstroke can strike at any time.[27] The cascade toward heat illness occurs when the body cannot facilitate adequate heat loss to maintain a normal core temperature. Mechanisms of evaporative cooling and vascular shunting to the extremities are overpowered by excessive heat production or high ambient temperatures.

Risk factors for heat-related illness include increasing age, obesity, ongoing infection, dehydration, alcohol consumption, use of anticholinergic, neuroleptic, stimulant, or diuretic medications, and comorbid medical conditions such as diabetes, sickle cell trait, and cardiovascular issues. Some individuals may be more prone to heat-related illness and have multiple recurrent episodes throughout their athletic career. Therefore, documentation of heat exhaustion or stroke is critical to prevent future occurrences.

Heat edema, rash, muscle cramping are the first signs of mild heat illness. As peripheral vasodilation occurs to facilitate heat transfer, fluid leaks into the interstitial space causing dependent soft tissue swelling. There may also be erythema or rash associated with this physiologic state. Heat cramps can occur as dehydration and electrolyte abnormalities progress, primarily affecting the large muscle groups in the abdomen and lower extremities. A growing body of evidence suggests that cramping is also the result of altered neuromuscular excitability, in which muscle fatigue and damage contribute to increased alpha motor neuron activity.[28]

Heat exhaustion is defined by a combination of symptoms such as nausea, vomiting, dizziness, irritability, headache, weakness, fatigability, muscle cramping, and decreased urinary output in the setting of high body temperatures between 101°F and 104°F. Exhaustion occurs when the demands of heat exchange, muscular exertion, and visceral organ function exceed cardiac output. As a result, athletes may have cold and clammy skin despite significant diaphoresis and elevated core body temperature. The most effective modality of treatment is removal from heat and sun exposure, removal of excessive clothing, and ice water immersion. Adjunctive therapies, such as fans and ice packs, may provide further symptomatic relief, but do not replace immersion. Importantly, athlete mental status should be continually monitored, as any signs of mental status change with elevated core temperature are indicative of heatstroke.

Unlike illness or exhaustion, heatstroke is a true medical emergency characterized by elevation of core body temperature above 105°F leading to altered mental status, systemic inflammatory response, and multiorgan failure.[29] Hot skin and hemodynamic instability are other key distinguishing factors from heat exhaustion. When cooling with ice water immersion is initiated within 30 minutes of symptom onset, mortality is exceedingly low.[30] However, prognosis is related to the duration of hyperthermia, as continued elevated core body temperature above 105°F more than 30 minutes leads to mortality rates approaching 80%.[29] Rectal temperature should be continuously monitored while in the acute cooling phase. A cold or ice water bath should always be made available, but immediate cooling by any means necessary should be pursued when submersion is not an option. Alternatives include drenching the athlete in cold water or using cold wet towels and sheets. Cold saline infusion can be used in addition to these measures when intravenous access is secured, as potential benefits exist in reducing hepatorenal injury.[31] Importantly, antipyretics or dantrolene are not useful for heatstroke.[32]

Emergency services should be summoned, although the athlete is initially stabilized and submersion therapy begins. Emergency personnel are recommended to cool the athlete on-field granted that appropriate treatments are available. Continued cooling measures during transport to the emergency department are essential. Even after resolution of elevated core temperature and normalization of mental status, patients are at risk of several other sequelae requiring hospital admission, including hepatorenal injury, electrolyte disturbances, rhabdomyolysis, pulmonary complications, and compartment syndrome.

There is limited evidence regarding safe return to sport after heat illness and heatstroke; however, the American College of Sports Medicine[33] indicates that athletes should refrain from exercise for at least 7 days after discharge from the hospital with 1-week follow-up for evaluation with relevant laboratory testing. Given normalization of laboratory markers and improved examination, the athlete may be cleared for slow progression to training with initial exercise taking place in a cool environment. At least 2 weeks should be required for outdoor training before return to competition.

SUDDEN CARDIAC ARREST

Sudden cardiac arrest in athletes is a rare but tragic event highly publicized among amateurs and professionals over the years. Screening tools and examinations for cardiovascular abnormalities have helped the sports medicine physician to better risk stratify and more safely govern athlete participation by primary prevention. In particular, the American Heart Association (AHA) has published pre-participation guidelines specific to athletes, consisting of a 14-point history and physical examination evaluating for risk of sudden cardiac arrest. The AHA screening components query whether an athlete has exertional chest pain, previous episodes syncope or near syncope, presence of a heart murmur, hypertension, family history of early cardiac death, cardiomyopathy, and examination signs consistent with coarctation or Marfan's syndrome. Evaluation with electrocardiography has also become standard for athlete screening to detect cardiovascular abnormalities which may not be evident by physical examination. Studies increasingly suggest that ECG screening added to history and physical (H&P) is more efficient and cost-effective at detecting conditions associated with sudden cardiac arrest in athletes. Clinicians should consider ECG screening as primary prevention for sudden cardiac arrest (SCA) and include if feasible for practice and secondary referral settings.[34,35]

The most common causes of sudden cardiac arrest categorized as electrical, acquired, or structural abnormalities. Hypertrophic cardiomyopathy, congenital coronary artery anomalies, Marfan's syndrome, arrhythmogenic right ventricular cardiomyopathy, or valvular dysfunction are the chief examples of structural abnormalities. Likewise, electrical cardiac abnormalities include Wolff–Parkinson–White syndrome, congenital long QT syndrome, and Brugada syndrome. Finally, acquired cardiac abnormalities consist of infection, trauma, toxicity, or environmental factors leading to dysrhythmias.

Care of the athlete with an identified cardiovascular abnormality via screening can be challenging, as many athletes are previously unaware of their diagnosis. Uncertainty may exist regarding training and competition protocols after diagnosis, especially in asymptomatic athletes. The AHA has published several iterations of consensus strategies to support the athlete while protecting them from severe complications.[36] These recommendations are organized by cardiovascular disease type. However, the AHA recommendations are based on expert opinion and afford the sports medicine physician an opportunity to deviate from recommendations given their personal evaluation of an athlete.

SUMMARY OF RECOMMENDATIONS

- A well-defined plan and systematic approach is the cornerstone of quality health care delivery as defined by the EAP.
- Team-based collaboration is necessary for the safety of the athlete and the success of the treatment plan; the skills of all team members must be leveraged.
- Emergency response preparation begins well before athletes take the field.
- In most instances, primary and secondary prevention strategies will lead to safe training and competition for athletes.

CLINICS CARE POINTS

- Emergency Action Plans (EAPs) should be developed and reviewed on an annual basis.
- A sports medicine emergency kit should cover routine medical events or injuries as well as tailored to sports-specific needs.
- The availability of regularly maintained automatic emergency defibrillators (AEDs) can lower the rate of death associated with sudden cardiac arrest.
- An athlete's medical history should be well-known and documented to prevent any potential emergencies associated with underlying endocrine, neurological, cardiopulmonary, and environmental disease or illness.

DISCLOSURE

The authors have no relevant commercial or financial information to disclose.

REFERENCES

1. McDermott ER, Tennent DJ, Patzkowski JC. On-field Emergencies and Emergency Action Plans. Sports Med Arthrosc Rev 2021;29(4):e51–6.
2. Long AM, Lefebvre CM, Mowery NT, et al. The Golden Opportunity: Multidisciplinary Simulation Training Improves Trauma Team Efficiency. J Surg Educ 2019;76(4):1116–21.
3. Ward KR. The microcirculation: linking trauma and coagulopathy. Transfusion 2013;53(Suppl 1):38s–47s.
4. Galicia-Garcia U, Benito-Vicente A, Jebari S, et al. Pathophysiology of Type 2 Diabetes Mellitus. Int J Mol Sci 2020;21(17).
5. Bussau VA, Ferreira LD, Jones TW, et al. The 10-s maximal sprint: a novel approach to counter an exercise-mediated fall in glycemia in individuals with type 1 diabetes. Diabetes Care 2006;29(3):601–6.
6. Shepherd PR, Kahn BB. Glucose transporters and insulin action–implications for insulin resistance and diabetes mellitus. N Engl J Med 1999;341(4):248–57.
7. Frid A, Ostman J, Linde B. Hypoglycemia risk during exercise after intramuscular injection of insulin in thigh in IDDM. Diabetes Care 1990;13(5):473–7.
8. Bognetti F., Brunelli A., Meschi F., et al., Frequency and correlates of severe hypoglycaemia in children and adolescents with diabetes mellitus, *Eur J Pediatr*, 156 (8), 1997, 589–591.
9. Kirk SE. Hypoglycemia in athletes with diabetes. Clin Sports Med 2009;28(3):455–68.
10. Jimenez C.C., Corcoran M.H., Crawley J.T., et al., National athletic trainers' association position statement: management of the athlete with type 1 diabetes mellitus, *J Athl Train*, 42 (4), 2007, 536–545.
11. MacDonald MJ. Postexercise late-onset hypoglycemia in insulin-dependent diabetic patients. Diabetes Care 1987;10(5):584–8.
12. Hough DO. Diabetes mellitus in sports. Med Clin North Am 1994;78(2):423–37.
13. Hirsch I.B., Marker J.C., Smith L.J., et al., Insulin and glucagon in prevention of hypoglycemia during exercise in humans, *Am J Physiol*, 260 (5 Pt 1), 1991, E695–E704.
14. Weiler JM, Layton T, Hunt M. Asthma in United States Olympic athletes who participated in the 1996 Summer Games. J Allergy Clin Immunol 1998;102(5):722–6.
15. Ross RG. The prevalence of reversible airway obstruction in professional football players. Med Sci Sports Exerc 2000;32(12):1985–9.
16. Anderson SD, Kippelen P. Exercise-induced bronchoconstriction: pathogenesis. Curr Allergy Asthma Rep 2005;5(2):116–22.
17. Fitch K.D., Sue-Chu M., Anderson S.D., et al., Asthma and the elite athlete: summary of the International Olympic Committee's consensus conference, Lausanne, Switzerland, January 22-24, 2008, *J Allergy Clin Immunol*, 122 (2), 2008, 254–260, 260.e1-7.
18. Boulet L-P, O'Byrne PM. Asthma and Exercise-Induced Bronchoconstriction in Athletes. N Engl J Med 2015;372(7):641–8.
19. Sue-Chu M. Winter sports athletes: long-term effects of cold air exposure. Br J Sports Med 2012;46(6):397–401.

20. Langdeau J.B., Turcotte H., Bowie D.M., et al., Airway hyperresponsiveness in elite athletes, *Am J Respir Crit Care Med*, 161 (5), 2000, 1479–1484.
21. Subbarao P, Duong M, Adelroth E, et al. Effect of ciclesonide dose and duration of therapy on exercise-induced bronchoconstriction in patients with asthma. J Allergy Clin Immunol 2006;117(5):1008–13.
22. Duong M., Amin R., Baatjes A.J., et al., The effect of montelukast, budesonide alone, and in combination on exercise-induced bronchoconstriction, *J Allergy Clin Immunol*, 130 (2), 2012, 535–539.e3.
23. Elkins MR, Brannan JD. Warm-up exercise can reduce exercise-induced bronchoconstriction. Br J Sports Med 2013;47(10):657–8.
24. Carter JM, McGrew C. Seizure Disorders and Exercise/Sports Participation. Curr Sports Med Rep 2021;20(1):26–30.
25. Lopes DM, McMahon SB. Ultraviolet Radiation on the Skin: A Painful Experience? CNS Neurosci Ther 2016;22(2):118–26.
26. Shih B.B., Farrar M.D., Cooke M.S., et al., Fractional Sunburn Threshold UVR Doses Generate Equivalent Vitamin D and DNA Damage in Skin Types I-VI but with Epidermal DNA Damage Gradient Correlated to Skin Darkness, *J Invest Dermatol*, 138 (10), 2018, 2244–2252.
27. Armstrong LE, Casa DJ, Millard-Stafford M, et al. Exertional Heat Illness during Training and Competition, Med Sci Sports Exerc 2007;39(3).
28. Miller KC. Rethinking the Cause of Exercise-Associated Muscle Cramping: Moving beyond Dehydration and Electrolyte Losses. Curr Sports Med Rep 2015;14(5).
29. Pryor R.R., Bennett B.L., O'Connor F.G., et al., Medical Evaluation for Exposure Extremes: Heat, *Wilderness Environ Med*, 26 (4 Suppl), 2015, S69–S75.
30. Sloan B.K., Kraft E.M., Clark D., et al., On-site treatment of exertional heat stroke, *Am J Sports Med*, 43 (4), 2015, 823–829.
31. Mok G, DeGroot D, Hathaway NE, et al. Exertional Heat Injury: Effects of Adding Cold (4°C) Intravenous Saline to Prehospital Protocol. Curr Sports Med Rep 2017; 16(2):103–8.
32. Lipman G.S., Gaudio F.G., Eifling K.P., et al., Wilderness Medical Society Clinical Practice Guidelines for the Prevention and Treatment of Heat Illness: 2019 Update, *Wilderness Environ Med*, 30 (4s), 2019, S33–S46.
33. O'Connor F.G., Casa D.J., BBergeron M.F., et al., American College of Sports Medicine Roundtable on exertional heat stroke–return to duty/return to play: conference proceedings, *Curr Sports Med Rep*, 9 (5), 2010, 314–321.
34. Harmon K.G., Suchsland M.Z., Prutkin J.M., et al., Comparison of cardiovascular screening in college athletes by history and physical examination with and without an electrocardiogram: Efficacy and cost, *Heart Rhythm*, 17 (10), 2020, 1649–1655.
35. Drezner J.A., Owens D.S., Prutkin J.M., et al., Electrocardiographic Screening in National Collegiate Athletic Association Athletes, *Am J Cardiol*, 118 (5), 2016, 754–759.
36. Maron BJ, Zipes DP, Kovacs RJ. Eligibility and Disqualification Recommendations for Competitive Athletes With Cardiovascular Abnormalities: Preamble, Principles, and General Considerations: A Scientific Statement From the American Heart Association and American College of Cardiology. J Am Coll Cardiol 2015;66(21):2343–9.

Heat, Cold, and Environmental Emergencies in Athletes

Kartik Sidhar, MD[a,*], Katlyn Elliott, MD[b], Michael Ibrahem, MD[c]

KEYWORDS

- Environment • Heat • Altitude • Sports • Hypothermia • Frostbite • Heatstroke

KEY POINTS

- Understand cold-related illness and recognize emergent management indications for frostbite, hypothermia, and nonfreezing injuries.
- Identify and understand heat-related illnesses including diagnosis and emergent management of heatstroke.
- Recognize signs and symptoms of altitude sickness and use appropriate diagnosis to guide management.

A survey completed in 2020 showed more than 160 million Americans participated in at least one outdoor activity.[1] Outdoor activities and sports lack a climate-controlled setting and protection from environmental elements resulting in unique risks to factor in when providing medical coverage for outdoor events. Prompt diagnosis and management of cold, heat, and other environmental-related illnesses or events can improve outcomes in the care of athletes.

EXERTIONAL HEAT ILLNESS

Severe weather conditions can make it difficult to practice and compete for athletes, particularly in excessive heat.[2] Heat illness can present anytime with extended strenuous exercise,[3] and it can manifest in a variety of ways ranging from mild symptoms, including heat edema, rash, cramps, syncope, to severe presentations including heatstroke (**Fig. 1**).[4] Prompt recognition and management can mitigate the progression to severe exertional heat illness and minimize morbidity and mortality.

---

[a] Department of Family Medicine, University of Michigan Medical School, 300 North Ingalls Street, NI4C06, Ann Arbor, MI 48109-5435, USA; [b] University of Pittsburgh Medical Center, McKeesport Family Medicine Residency, 2347 5th Avenue, McKeesport, PA 15132, USA; [c] University of Pittsburgh Medical Center, Shadyside Family Medicine Residency, 5215 Center Avenue, Pittsburgh, PA 15232, USA
* Corresponding author.
E-mail address: ksidhar@med.umich.edu

Clin Sports Med 42 (2023) 441–461
https://doi.org/10.1016/j.csm.2023.02.008
0278-5919/23/© 2023 Elsevier Inc. All rights reserved.

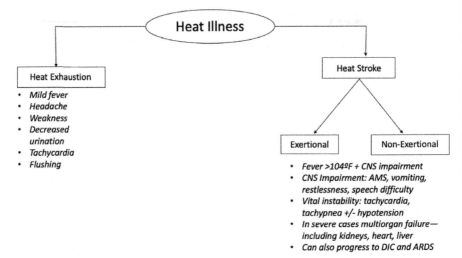

Fig. 1. Summary of heat-related injuries.

Heat Exhaustion

Clinical findings

Heat exhaustion can affect a wide variety of athletes, but the extremes of age groups are more vulnerable to injury.[5] Symptoms of heat exhaustion are nonspecific and include mild fever, nausea, fatigue, headaches, dizziness, and weakness.[6] Athletes may also present with decreased urination, flushing, and tachycardia.[6] Neurologic symptoms including confusion, syncope should prompt evaluation for more serious heat illnesses including heatstroke.[6]

Management

First steps in management include discontinuation of exercise, eliminating heat exposure, and removal of clothing or any material that might prevent heat dispersal.[7] Cooling the body by submerging or showering in cool water has been shown to improve outcomes.[7] Elevating legs can also improve blood return and alleviate orthostatic symptoms.[7] Prompt oral hydration, if possible, or IV hydration in those who cannot tolerate oral intake, is essential.[7] The athlete should be evaluated for heatstroke if the symptoms fail to ameliorate in 20 to 30 minutes after initiating the treatment or if patient meets temperature criteria in combination with neurologic symptoms as described below.[7]

Exertional Heatstroke

Heatstroke is a medical emergency and can be fatal[8] and has resulted in 39 deaths between 2000 and 2012 in football players including youth, high school, college, and professional football players.[9] In the United States, 3332 people died of heatstroke between 2006 and 2010.[10] Heatstroke is categorized as non-exertional, which is common in older individuals or exertional.[11] The focus of this review will be on exertional heat stroke (EHS) as it is one of the three leading causes of sudden death in athletes.[12] EHS can develop during the first hour after initiating physical exercise and is not necessarily dependent on the environmental temperature.[11] Aside from practicing in hot, humid weather, other risk factors include inadequate rest intervals, inappropriate attire, medications (diuretics, anti-depressants, antihistamines), stimulants, obesity, fever,[13] and overexertion.[11] Prompt recognition and immediate treatment can decrease morbidity and mortality.

Clinical findings
Diagnostic criteria include hyperthermia greater than 104°F along with central nervous system (CNS) impairment.[10] CNS symptoms may present as vomiting, altered mental status including decreased level of consciousness, speech difficulties, and restlessness.[11] Patients can present with tachycardia, tachypnea, or hypotension as well as excessive sweating or paradoxically dry hot skin in the setting of dehydration.[11] Untreated heatstroke can lead to multiorgan failure secondary to systemic inflammatory reaction which can involve the kidneys, heart, liver, muscles (rhabdomyolysis), and in extreme scenarios, disseminated intravascular coagulation and acute respiratory distress syndrome.[11]

Diagnosis/differential diagnosis
Clinical presentation is the cornerstone of diagnosis.[11] Checking rectal temperature is imperative and should be done as soon as heatstroke is suspected as late or improper measurement can delay treatment.[11] However, the isolated elevation of core temperature without other signs or symptoms as outlined above is not sufficient to establish a diagnosis of heatstroke.[11]

Treatment
Once the diagnosis of EHS is made, begin by initiating the emergency response system to ensure timely transportation (**Fig. 2**). This is especially important in remote trail races or events. The purpose of initial EHS treatment is to mitigate hyperthermia as soon as possible before transportation to decrease morbidity and mortality.[11,14] In general, a goal temperature of less than 102.5°F within 30 minutes of diagnosis, with a cooling rate around 0.37°F per minute, is recommended.[11] Cold water immersion (CWI) is the most effective method to drop body core temperature,[14] with a cooling rate of around 0.37°F per minute per minute.[11] Shaking, restlessness, and irritability can be associated with CWI rapid cooling, but will not affect the end result.[15] Other cooling methods include cool air exposure, a cool water spray, cooling blankets or towels, and ice packs to axilla, groin, and neck, where the large vessels are located.[14] Sometimes cooling methods are not enough,[11] and securing the airway, maintaining blood pressure with IV fluids, and vasopressors may be necessary.[15] It is also worth mentioning that administering oral fluids could be risky in patients with compromised mentation.[16] Antipyretics are not indicated due to the lack of efficacy and the risk of exacerbating hepatopathy and coagulopathy.[11]

Outcomes/prevention
Mortality is generally low (<5%) as EHS usually occurs in younger healthy athletes.[11] Regardless, EHS remains one of the three leading causes of death in athletes.[12] It is thought the duration rather than degree of hyperthermia is associated with morbidity and mortality.[17] Therefore, early diagnosis and rapid initiation of cooling is key in management. If temperature is brought to below 104°F within 30 minutes of onset of neurologic symptoms, mortality approaches zero.[12]

Prevention strategies include acclimatization to new weather conditions, avoiding the hottest hours of the day, matching practice load to fitness level, incorporating structured breaks, maintaining hydration status, and wearing appropriate attire.[11] A helpful tool to predict risk of heat injury is the wet bulb globe temperature which integrates ambient temperature, wind speed, solar radiation, and most importantly, humidity.[2]

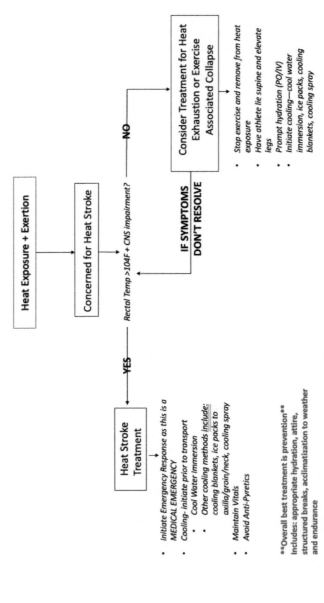

Fig. 2. Diagnosis and treatment algorithm for heat-related illness.

EXERCISE-ASSOCIATED COLLAPSE (HEAT SYNCOPE)

Exercise-associated collapse (EAC), which was previously known as heat syncope, is usually encountered following cessation of vigorous activity.[18] EAC can be related to factors including high ambient temperature, dehydration, hyponatremia, or hypoglycemia.[19] Pathophysiology of EAC is thought to be due to pooling of the blood in the lower extremities.[20] The subsequent heat/fluid depletion causes cardiovascular stress[21] and orthostatic hypotension.[22] EAC presents as dizziness, difficulty standing/ambulating, and/or syncope,[20] without loss of consciousness.[23] Although EAC is a benign event, it should be distinguished from other serious exertion-related illnesses as it could have similar presentation.[22]

Management of EAC in normothermic patients should include placing patients in supine position with elevated legs to treat postural hypotension.[22] Additional evaluation is warranted if mentation has not returned to baseline after 5 minutes or if vital sign instability occurs,[22] as these findings can be indicative of EHS.[20] Finally, EAC should be distinguished from exercise-related syncope, which occurs during exercise and is more likely related to concerning underlying cardiac etiology.[19]

Cold-Related Illness

Between 2006 and 2010, two-thirds of all weather-related deaths in the United States were associated with excessive cold.[24] These injuries occur year-round during physical activity in the setting of low air temperatures, low water temperatures, windy conditions, or a combination of these circumstances. According to national data, approximately 3% to 5% of all injuries in mountaineers and up to 20% in Nordic skiing are due to hypothermia or frostbite.[24] Cold illnesses can be broken down into three categories: hypothermia, freezing injuries, and nonfreezing injuries (**Fig. 3**). Factors that increase a person's risk of sustaining a cold injury are broken down into environmental risk factors, non-environmental risk factors, and medical conditions/medications (**Table 1**).

Accidental Hypothermia

Winter sports place athletes at risk for hypothermia and subsequent complications related to hypothermia. Sports at risk include cold weather events, especially longer exposure endurance events including cross-country skiing, running, triathlons, and other mountain sports.[25–27] Prevention and rapid diagnosis can decrease morbidity and mortality associated with hypothermia.

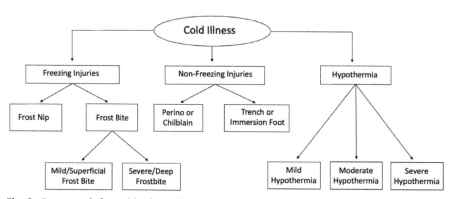

Fig. 3. Framework for cold-related illness.

Table 1
Summary of risk factors for cold injury[32]

Environmental Risk Factors	Non-Environmental Risk Factors	Medical Conditions	Medications
Wind chill	Previous cold injury	Asthma/COPD	Benzodiazepines
Precipitation	Low-caloric intake	Anorexia nervosa	Barbiturates
Lack of cold acclimatization	Dehydration	Cold urticaria	Cocaine, opioids, LSD, marijuana, amphetamines
Geographic regions which predispose to cold injury	Fatigue/exhaustion	Raynaud's	Clonidine
High altitude	Outdoor enthusiasts/athletes/workers	Cardiovascular disease; CAD, PVD, CHF	TCAs/MAOIs
High humidity	Constrictive clothing	Alcohol use disorder, polysubstance use disorder	Nicotine
Prolonged exposure	Aerobic fitness level/endurance	Diabetes	Insulin
	Inappropriate clothing/equipment	Hypothyroidism	Sulfonylurea's
	Age; young and old	Skin conditions: sunburns, psoriasis, hyperhidrosis	Anti-HTN meds
		Adrenal insufficiency	Beta blockers
		Hypopituitarism	Alcohol
		MS/Parkinson's/spinal cord injury	Antihistamines
		Dementia	Laxatives

Abbreviations: CAD, coronary artery disease; CHF, congestive heart failure; COPD, chronic obstructive pulmonary disease; HTN, hypertension; LSD, lysergic acid diethylamide; MAOI, monoamine oxidase inhibitors; MS, multiple sclerosis; PVD, peripheral vascular disease; TCA, tricyclic antidepressant.

Clinical findings

Criteria for hypothermia are met when core body temperature is less than 95°F.[24] Severity ranges from mild, moderate, or severe based on core body temperature. Each category of hypothermia is associated with signs and symptoms that can aid in diagnosis and guide management.[28]

Signs and symptoms

Mild hypothermia (89.6°F–95°F). Mild hypothermia presents with vague symptoms including fatigue and nausea. Systemic responses include hypertension, tachycardia, and tachypnea to assist with passive heating.[29] Additional symptoms include a decrease in cognitive function and decision-making as well as increased urination.[30]

Moderate hypothermia (82.4°F–89.6°F). The main symptom to differentiate from mild hypothermia is progressive cognitive decline. Additional symptoms include hypotension, bradycardia, and cessation of shivering at 86°F to 89.6 F. Some individuals may paradoxically begin removing layers of clothing which can delay diagnosis of hypothermia.[31]

Severe hypothermia (<82.4°F). Individuals have increased susceptibility to arrhythmias and a decrease in brain perfusion. An athlete may become unconscious and sustain cardiopulmonary arrest.[30]

Evaluation and management

Prompt, on-field evaluation can help diagnose mild hypothermia and prevent progression and complications associated with moderate and severe hypothermia. Evaluation with history and physical to assess mental status along with obtaining an accurate, preferably, rectal temperature in individuals of concern is necessary to adequately categorize severity of hypothermia.[30]

Treatment

The best methods for rewarming vary based on the severity of hypothermia. In a limited, on-field, setting, most options would include passive rewarming. For mild hypothermia, begin by removing wet clothing and remove the athlete from cold exposure if possible. Begin passive rewarming strategies including hot packs to axillary regions and application of heated blankets.[32] Add glucose-containing warmed beverages to provide energy for shivering and avoid using friction such as rubbing cool extremities as this can increase tissue trauma.[33]

For moderate and severe hypothermia, continue passive warming while in the field as above. Addition of external warming methods including warm air can be added. If able, heated IV fluids can be added for rewarming. Consider adding oral or IV glucose as discussed above to provide energy for shivering which can greatly assist with rewarming.[30] Higher risk of cardiac arrhythmias is present at temperatures lower than 89.6 F, so continue to monitor vitals and maintain a high level of suspicious for cardiac arrest if athlete has changes in mental status.[32] Initiate prompt transfer to higher level of care, especially if event is in a remote or a high-altitude setting with unpredictable weather.

Prevention

Cold injury prevention recommendations according to the American College of Sports Medicine include:[34]

1. Coaches/athletes/medical personnel:
   - Aware of the signs and symptoms of cold injuries
     ○ Hypothermia

- ○ Frostbite
- ○ Nonfreezing cold injuries
- • Identify individuals susceptible to cold injuries
- • Have updated information regarding weather conditions
2. Clothing
   - • Chosen based on individual
   - • Standardized clothing not necessary
3. Wind chill
   - • Wind chill temperature index to measure risk of frostbite
   - • Increased monitoring when wind-chill temperatures are below −17°F

Nonfreezing Cold Injury

Nonfreezing injuries occur when cold exposure leads to cellular damage without formation of ice crystals. The two most common injuries within this category include immersion/trench foot and chilblain/pernio.

Immersion/trench foot

Immersion/trench foot is a nonfreezing injury that occurs with prolonged exposure, typically between 12 and 96 hours, to wet conditions with temperatures above 32°F. The typical mechanism of injury involves continued exposure to wet socks/footwear.[35] This results in increased absorption of moisture leading to high levels of extracellular fluid which causes inflammation and peripheral vasoneuropathy.[35–37] Additional risk factors include the presence of trauma, malnutrition, exhaustion, infection, lymphedema, or venous hypertension.[35]

Clinical findings

Immersion/trench foot typically presents as numbness, burning, or tingling sensation which occurs before affected area is removed from the cold exposure. After removed from exposure, skin typically becomes mottled while the numbness and burning sensation intensifies.[35] Eventually, skin becomes edematous and is associated with a variety of lesions including blisters, fissures, and maceration.[35,36,38,39]

Treatment

If immersion/trench foot is suspected, move athlete to a warm dry place. Evaluate for hypothermia and frostbite. After these conditions have been excluded or treated appropriately,[35] the affected foot should be thoroughly cleaned and dried. After this, rewarm with warm packs or soaking in warm water (102°F–110°F) for approximately 5 minutes.[35–39] Affected foot should be elevated and allowed to dry at room temperature. Advise the athlete to avoid weight bearing as this has been shown to be improve healing.[39] Immersion/trench foot is associated with intense pain at onset of injury as well as on rewarming which must be addressed. Trials have shown improved pain control with amitriptyline when compared with nonsteroidal anti-inflammatory (NSAIDs) or opioids.[40]

Outcomes/prevention

If not treated appropriately, immersion/trench foot can be complicated by cellulitis, sepsis, and cellular necrosis which can lead to amputation.[35] After the limb is rewarmed, a post-injury phase involving sensorimotor and autonomic deficits can be present from weeks to years.[37]

Overall, the best treatment of immersion/trench foot is prevention.[38] This can be done through education regarding appropriate equipment and maintaining a dry environment through waterproof boots, moisture wicking socks, frequent sock/foot-wear changes, and rotation of wet footwear to prevent immersion/trench foot.[36–38]

Chilblain/Pernio

Chilblain/pernio is a nonfreezing injury which is characterized by localized inflamma-tory lesions that predominately affect hands and feet within 24 hours after prolonged exposure to cold or damp environments.[36,41] The severity of chilblain/pernio depends on both duration of exposure and temperature during exposure.[41] The pathophysi-ology of chilblain/pernio is not well understood but hypothesized to be secondary to hypoxemic vasospasm of affected tissue in the setting of prolonged cold exposure.[42]

Clinical presentation

Risk factors for development of chilblain/pernio include all general risk factors for cold injuries but special attention should be paid to athletes with a history of systemic lupus erythematosus (SLE).[43]

Chilblain typically presents as symmetrically distributed erythematous papules or ulcers in extremities after cold exposure.[39] These lesions are associated with a variety of sensations including tenderness, itching, tingling, burning, and increased edema and warmth over the affected area.[36,41,42] Unlike frostbite, skin necrosis and tissue loss are uncommon.[42] Symptoms may come and go. Symptom onset typically occurs in the winter and single episodes can last up to 1 to 3 weeks with spontaneous reso-lution, although annual occurrences are common.[42]

Treatment

Management involves removal of wet/constrictive clothing, washing and gently drying affected area and elevation of affected area followed by rewarming by covering affected extremities with loose dry blanket.[42] Throughout the rewarming process, continual evaluation of sensation and circulation return is critical. Return of sensation, temperature, and circulation can lead to pain in the affected area which should be treatment with appropriate analgesia.[44] Avoid disrupting blisters, minimize friction, and discourage weight bearing on affected extremity.[36,37,44,45] After the athlete is removed from exposure and rewarming has been started, pharmacologic therapy with nifedipine can be initiated which acts as a vasodilator and can improve the episode as well as prevent recurrence.[44] Given the potential association, the presence of chilblains should prompt a screen for SLE.[43,46] Overall data regarding medical treat-ment of chilblains limited, but the best treatment is prevention and education.[38]

Outcomes

Despite relapsing and remitting nature of this condition, the prognosis of chilblains/pernio is good and there is minimal functional impairment or long-term complica-tions.[42] Given the possible association with rheumatologic disorders, workup or referral for evaluation is indicated.[46]

Freezing Cold-Related Injury

If cold stress continues, tissues freeze, resulting in crystallization within tissue which occurs only when temperatures fall below 37°F.[47] One of the major groups at risk of freezing injuries includes mountaineers. One study found the incidence of freezing injury in mountaineer's was 366/1000 population per year.[27] Other groups which expe-rience freezing cold injuries include Nordic and Alpine skiers.[26]

Frostbite

There are three distinct phases of frostbite which include frostnip or pre-freeze phase, mild frostbite, or the freeze-thaw phase and finally severe frostbite or deep freeze

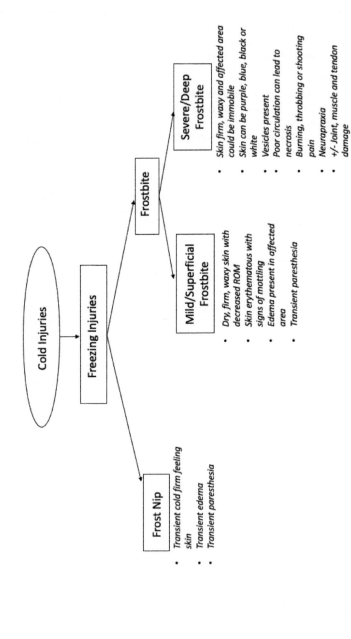

Fig. 4. Summary of freezing cold injury and typical presentations. ROM, range of motion.

phase (**Fig. 4**). These phases are delineated by the extent of cyanosis present after rewarming and depth of tissue affected.[32]

Frostnip

Frostnip is a freezing injury which is considered a mild precursor to frostbite in which superficial cell layer freezes without permanent damage. It is termed the "pre-freeze" which can occur if superficial skin cools to 37°F to 50°F.[24] Like in all cold injuries, frostnip most often seen in peripheral tissue especially the face and extremities. Frostnip presents as transient hyperesthesia/paresthesia and edema that often self-limiting and resolve within 10 minutes of rewarming or removal from cold exposure.[38] As with all other cold injuries, the development of frostnip may cause athletes to become more sensitive to cold in the future. Athletes with a history of frostnip or frostbite are two to four times more likely to develop frostbite in the same area again.[48] This typically corresponds to Grade 1 frostbite after rewarming.

Mild/superficial frostbite

As tissue temperature reaches 5°F to 21°F intra, extracellular ice crystals begin to form which leads to cell rupture and subsequent crystallization.[36] This process is termed the "freeze-thaw phase" and typically involves surrounding skin, adjacent vasculature, nerves, and subcutaneous tissue.[49] Individuals often present with dry/waxy erythematous and edematous skin.[32,49] The involved skin area feels cold and firm to touch. There may be stiffness, decreased mobility of affected area, and burning sensation, which is exacerbated on rewarming.[49,50] Lesions are unlikely to blister at this stage,[50] but it is possible. Mild/superficial frostbite typically corresponds to Grade II frostbite after rewarming.

Severe/deep frostbite

Severe or deep frostbite involves the "venous stasis" phase which involves ice crystal formation leading to vasospasm and stasis coagulation.[36] As the cold exposure persists or tissue temperatures drops less than 5°F, injury progresses to the "ischemic" phase which is characterized by ischemia, gangrene, thrombosis, and autonomic dysfunction.[36,50] The tissue involvement of severe frostbite extends into muscles, tendons, deeper nerve structures, and even bone. This stress often leads to muscle, nerve, joint damage and in younger athletes can lead to premature closure of the epiphyseal plate.[49] Typically, severe/deep frostbite corresponds to Grade III/IV frostbite after rewarming.

Frostbite classification, evaluation, and management

An athlete who is being worked up for potential frostbite should first be removed from cold stress and an evaluation for hypothermia should be completed (**Fig. 5**).[32] In the field, remove wet and constrictive clothing and consider splinting/padding the involved limb if necessary for stabilization. Avoid manipulating blisters or weight-bearing on affected area as this can increase tissue damage. Rewarming should be avoided during transport if there is a chance of refreezing as the cycle of refreezing has been associated with significantly increased morbidity and tissue damage.[32] Once patient is in a warm location, rapid rewarming protocol can begin with the goal of enhancing tissue viability (**Table 2**). Rapid rewarming ideally done in whirlpool with water temperature of 98.6°F to 104°F and any form of dry heat is not recommended.[49] The rewarming process usually takes 15 to 30 minutes but is completed when tissue becomes soft and red/purple color.[24,32,49] During the rewarming process, most patients experience significant pain and appropriate analgesia is indicated.[50]

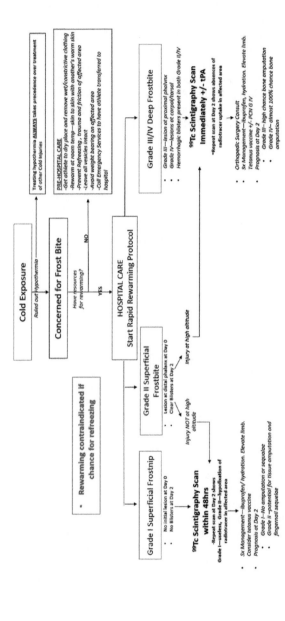

Fig. 5. Evaluation and treatment algorithm for frostbite.[32,77,78]

Table 2
In-field and hospital treatment of frostbite[32,77]

Prehospital Rewarming Protocol	Hospital Rapid Rewarming Protocol
Get athlete to dry place and remove wet/constrictive clothing	Patients with acute frostbite should be hospitalized
Rewarm at room temperature—skin to skin with another's warm skin	On admission, rewarming in warm water bath (98°F–104°F) for 15–30 min or until tissue softens or becomes red/purple.
Prevent refreezing, trauma, and friction of affected area. Avoid weight bearing on affected area.	Determine severity of frostbite based on cyanosis and other clinical symptoms. Perform ^{99}Tc scintigraphy scan ± tPA
Wound care: Leave all vesicles intact	Wound care: Debride white/hypopigmented blisters. Leave hemorrhagic blisters alone. Topical aloe applied to blisters. No occlusive dressings.
Pain management: Ibuprofen	Pain Management: Ibuprofen ± Morphine
Call emergency services to have athlete transferred to hospital	Infection control: Administer anti-tetanus prophylaxis ± IV Penicillin G within the first 24–72 h

Frostbite classification occurs after rewarming and is graded I–IV (**Fig. 6, Table 3**).[49] Frostbite is an injury that continues to progress over time with edema noted within 3 hours, vesicles within 6 hours, eschar within 9 days, and mummification of tissue within 22 days.[32,49] Management ranges from conservative management for mild cases to tissue plasminogen activator and possible debridement/amputation in severe cases.[49] If there is evidence of gangrene, delayed debridement/amputation is preferred as time is necessary to confirm demarcated borders of viable and necrotic tissue.[49]

Other complications of frostbite include scarring, nail damage, vasospasm on exposure to cold and increased likelihood of subsequent cold injury, hyperesthesia /hypoesthesia of involved area, chronic pain, peripheral neuropathy, and decreased proprioception after the event.[49] Athletes may also experience frostbite osteoarthritis,

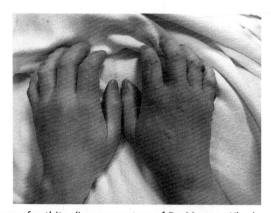

Fig. 6. Second-degree frostbite. (Image courtesy of Dr. Morteza Khodaee.)

Table 3
Frostbite classification after rewarming[77]

Frostbite Injuries	Grade I	Grade II	Grade III	Grade IV
Extent of injury at day 0 after rewarming	No initial lesion	Initial lesions at distal phalanx	Initial lesion at proximal phalanx	Initial lesion at carpal or tarsal
Bone scan at day 2	No findings	Hypofixation of radiotracer in affected area	Absence of radiotracer in affected area	Absence of radiotracer in affected area
Blisters at day 2	None	Clear blisters	Hemorrhagic blisters	Hemorrhagic blisters
Prognosis at day 2	No amputation	Tissue amputation	Bone amputation	Bone amputation ± systemic involvement ± sepsis

which is characterized by joint swelling, transient flexion contracture, and joint damage in hands.[50] In the pediatric population, one serious complication is premature closure of epiphyseal plate with subsequent growth abnormality.[51] Unfortunately, no treatment has been shown to prevent permanent bone and joint sequelae in children.[51]

Overall, the best treatment for cold injuries is prevention and preparation.[34] The summary of necessary preparations to actively prevent cold injury is listed in **Box 1**.

EXTREME WEATHER-RELATED EMERGENCIES
Lightning

Lightning strikes results in approximately 27 deaths per year with around 270 nonfatal lightning strikes per year.[52] Most of the lightning strikes occur during the day between April and September.[53] This timing, unfortunately, correlates with timing of many outdoor sporting events. Previous epidemiologic data showed soccer had the highest incidence of lightning-related fatalities followed by golf and running.[54]

Diagnosis and management
Initial evaluation after lightning strike should entail a brief history and physical examination looking for signs of lightning strike. Lightning strike can result in tissue injury from thermal damage or electrical abnormality of the heart resulting in asystole or arrhythmia resulting in sudden cardiac death.[55] Management of lightning strike victims should be completed using a "reverse triage" as those with sudden cardiac and respiratory arrest should be addressed first.[55] Many will have spontaneous return of rhythm but will require respiratory support.

Flash Flood

Although tornadoes and hurricanes are notorious for causing significant devastation and mortality, flash floods are a leading cause of weather-related deaths in the United

---

Box 1
Summary of necessary preparations to actively prevent cold injury

Cold Injury Prevention

- Education on appropriate clothing/equipment
  - Loose layered clothing; ideally base layer allows for sweat evaporation with minimal absorption, middle layer can wick moisture and provides insulation as well as an outer layer is water/wind resistant while allowing for some ventilation.
  - Removal of wet socks/footwear with frequent changes at appropriate intervals to allow for drying
  - Trial of equipment before activity to ensure it is functional
- Understanding of demands of activity and appropriate preparation
  - Proper conditioning before, during, and after event/activity
  - Be aware of situations which lead to exhaustion, stress, or excessive sweating and take appropriate breaks
  - Preparation of all necessary fluid/caloric intake needed for activity
- Event Contingency Planning
  - Ensure event has developed risk management guidelines which can be used to make decisions about participation in specific conditions—rain, wind chill, extreme cold.
  - Identify high-risk individuals/populations
  - Ensure all coaches, training staff, medical staff are educated on signs and symptoms of cold injuries and treatment guidelines
  - Ensure event center has appropriate equipment to manage cold injuries and capability to contact emergency personal if needed

States.[56,57] Between 2012 and 2021, there have been over 100 flood-related deaths per year in the United States. Many of these are related to driving in flooded streets.[58] However, with the an increase in mountaineering sports and public interest in hiking, flood-related deaths while in national and state recreation areas have also risen, specifically with an increase in deaths in the southwest where slot canyons are more prevalent.[59–61]

Prevention is the best method to prevent flood-related deaths. Advise athletes to monitor weather conditions and seek advice from the national weather service and national parks services when going into high-risk flash flood regions.[62] If an athlete is stuck in a situation with an impending flash flood, advise to get to the highest ground possible and avoid slot canyons. Coordination with national park rangers and local search and rescue before events can lead to improved and more effective disaster response.

ALTITUDE-RELATED ILLNESS
Acute Mountain Sickness

Acute mountain sickness (AMS) typically occurs at altitudes greater than 8000 feet.[63] The incidence of AMS is likely to increase given the rise in climbing sports in the United States with close to a twofold increase in climbing participants over the past decade.[64] Rapid diagnosis and treatment can prevent potentially life-threatening complications associated with altitude exposure.

Clinical findings and diagnosis

AMS in non-acclimatized individuals approaches around 75% above around 10,000 feet.[65] Symptoms usually begin a few hours after arriving at altitudes greater than 8000 feet. Clinical presentation is often vague. Symptoms may include headache, fatigue, light headedness, sleep disturbance, nausea, and/or vomiting. Headache tends to be the most common presenting symptom.[66] Pulse oximetry levels tend to be lower than normal reference ranges for a given altitude. Diagnosis is often clinical based on history and timing of exposure to high altitude.

Treatment and prevention

Mitigation strategies include slowing the rate of ascent to allow the body to adjust to reduced available oxygen at lower partial pressures.[65] Recommend limiting the rate of ascent to around 1500 feet per day at altitudes over 8000 feet with incorporated rest days every 3 to 4 days.[67,68] Experienced climbers may be more aware of their own limitations and time needed to acclimatize. Hypoxia exposure during sleep has not been shown to adequately decrease rates or symptoms associated with AMS.[69] Consider prophylaxis with acetazolamide if there is not adequate time to acclimatize or with high-altitude ascents.[67] Prophylaxis with acetazolamide has been shown to reduce the risk of AMS by 44%.[70] If the athlete cannot tolerate acetazolamide, consider dexamethasone for prophylaxis. Before using a steroid, ensure the athlete's sport will allow dexamethasone use as it is prohibited in competition by the World Anti-Doping Agency.[71]

In the athlete who has developed symptoms consistent with AMS, treatment includes discontinuing ascent and supportive care including NSAIDs, acetaminophen, and antiemetics for nausea. Depending on severity, acetazolamide or dexamethasone may be used for treatment.[66] Consider descent if symptoms are severe or do not resolve within a few days.

Complications of high-altitude exposure

High-altitude pulmonary edema. High altitude exposure and hypoxia causes pulmonary vasoconstriction which can lead to breakdown in the alveolar capillary barrier in the lungs leading to pulmonary effusion.[72] Untreated high-altitude pulmonary edema (HAPE) can result in up to 50% mortality. This condition more commonly affects healthy young males. The main distinguishing characteristics include hypoxia, cough, shortness of breath at rest, and decreased exercise tolerance.[72] Treatment involves descent of 3000 feet or until resolution of symptoms, supplemental oxygen, and portable hyperbaric chambers if descent is not possible. Nifedipine can be used as an adjunct as this decreases pulmonary vasoconstriction.[73] Prevention strategies include gradual ascent and nifedipine for prophylaxis.[74]

High-altitude cerebral edema. Another life-threatening complication of severe altitude exposure is high-altitude cerebral edema (HACE). Etiology is thought to be due to hypoxia-induced vasoconstriction similar to HAPE. Elevated capillary pressure from vasoconstriction leads to cerebral edema from disruption of the blood brain barrier.[75] Common symptoms can overlap with AMS including headache, fatigue, and nausea. Distinguishing features for HAPE include ataxia and altered mental status. Rapid diagnosis and treatment are imperative to prevent mortality from increased intracranial pressure. Treatment includes descent of around 3000 feet or until symptoms resolve, supplemental oxygen, or hyperbaric chamber if descent is not possible. Dexamethasone should be added as an adjunct for treatment of HACE.[76] Acetazolamide has less definitive evidence in the treatment of HACE but can be considered. Prevention includes gradual rate of ascent as described above and dexamethasone/acetazolamide can be used for prophylaxis.[75]

Outcomes/long-term recommendations
Outcomes for AMS are favorable and the majority will make a full recovery with descent and medication management as described above. Some may have persistent symptoms for 2 to 5 days. Rarely, symptoms may progress to more life-threatening illness including HACE and HAPE. If treated quickly and appropriately, HACE and HAPE can also have favorable outcomes. Prevention is preferred when appropriate and able.

SUMMARY

Outdoor sports can result in unique challenges from environmental exposures. The best strategy to mitigate heat, cold, climate, or altitude-related emergencies is proper counseling and prevention. If prevention is not possible, prompt recognition and initiation of appropriate management can lead to improved morbidity and mortality outcomes.

CLINICS CARE POINTS

- Exertional heatstroke is a medical emergency and requires prompt diagnosis and immediate treatment with cold water immersion.

- When evaluating cold injuries, evaluate and treat for hypothermia before addressing other extremity-related injuries.

- Delayed tissue debridement and amputation after frostbite leads to greater tissue preservation.

- Altitude exposure can lead to pulmonary edema or cerebral edema which are medical emergencies requiring rapid descent to decrease morbidity and mortality.

- Harsh climate exposure including lightning strikes and flash floods require appropriate event planning and response coordination.

DISCLOSURES

The authors have nothing to disclose.

REFERENCES

1. Executive Summary The Next Generation Outdoor Participation Snapshot A Detailed Look Participant Profile Methodology Diversity. Available at: Website 2021-Outdoor-Participation-Trends-Report.pdf (outdoorindustry.org). Accessed August 3, 2022.
2. Noonan B, Bancroft RW, Dines JS, et al. Heat- and Cold-induced Injuries in Athletes: Evaluation and Management. J Am Acad Orthop Surg 2012;20(12):744–54.
3. Armstrong LE, Casa DJ, Millard-Stafford M, et al. Exertional Heat Illness during Training and Competition. Med Sci Sports Exerc 2007;39(3):556–72.
4. Howe AS, Boden BP. Heat-Related Illness in Athletes. Am J Sports Med 2007; 35(8):1384–95.
5. Kenny GP, Wilson TE, Flouris AD, et al. Heat exhaustion. Handb Clin Neurol 2018;505–29.
6. Glazer JL. Management of heatstroke and heat exhaustion. Am Fam Physician 2005;71(11):2133–40. Available at: http://www.ncbi.nlm.nih.gov/pubmed/ 15952443.
7. Kenny GP, Wilson TE, Flouris AD, et al. Heat exhaustion. Handb Clin Neurol 2018;505–29.
8. Pryor RR, Roth RN, Suyama J, et al. Exertional Heat Illness: Emerging Concepts and Advances in Prehospital Care. Prehospital Disaster Med 2015;30(3): 297–305.
9. Schultz J, Kenney WL, Linden AD. Heat-Related Deaths in American Football: An Interdisciplinary Approach. Sport Hist Rev 2014;45(2):123–44.
10. Hifumi T, Kondo Y, Shimizu K, et al. Heat stroke. J Intensive Care 2018;6(1):30.
11. Epstein Y, Yanovich R, Heatstroke, et al, editors. N Engl J Med 2019;380(25): 2449–59.
12. Navarro CS, Casa DJ, Belval LN, et al. Exertional heat stroke. Curr Sports Med Rep 2017;16(5):304–5.
13. Navarro CS, Casa DJ, Belval LN, et al. Exertional Heat Stroke. Curr Sports Med Rep 2017;16(5):304–5.
14. Sloan BK, Kraft EM, Clark D, et al. On-Site Treatment of Exertional Heat Stroke. Am J Sports Med 2015;43(4):823–9.
15. Gaudio FG, Grissom CK. Cooling Methods in Heat Stroke. J Emerg Med 2016; 50(4):607–16.
16. Peiris AN, Jaroudi S, Noor R. Heat Stroke. JAMA 2017;318(24):2503.
17. Casa DJ, Armstrong LE, Kenny GP, et al. Exertional heat stroke: new concepts regarding cause and care. Curr Sports Med Rep 2012;11(3):115–23.
18. Gauer R, Meyers BK. Heat-Related Illnesses. Am Fam Physician 2019;99(8): 482–9.
19. Christou GA, Christou KA, Kiortsis DN. Pathophysiology of Noncardiac Syncope in Athletes. Sports Med 2018;48(7):1561–73.
20. Asplund CA, O'Connor FG, Noakes TD. Exercise-associated collapse: an evidence-based review and primer for clinicians. Br J Sports Med 2011;45(14): 1157–62.
21. Kenefick RW, Sawka MN. Heat Exhaustion and Dehydration as Causes of Marathon Collapse. Sports Med 2007;37(4):378–81.

22. Irelan MC, Schroeder JD. Exercise Associated Collapse. [Updated 2023 Jan 2]. In: StatPearls [Internet]. Treasure Island (FL): StatPearls Publishing; 2023. https://www.ncbi.nlm.nih.gov/books/NBK576425/.

23. Christou GA, Christou KA, Kiortsis DN. Pathophysiology of Noncardiac Syncope in Athletes. Sports Med 2018;48(7):1561–73.

24. Danzl DF, Pozos RS. Accidental Hypothermia. N Engl J Med 1994;113(20): 2579–82.

25. Smith M, Matheson GO, Meeuwisse WH. Injuries in cross-country skiing: a critical appraisal of the literature. Sports Med 1996;21(3):239–50.

26. Gammons M, Boynton M, Russell J, et al. On-mountain coverage of competitive skiing and snowboarding events. Curr Sports Med Rep 2011;10(3):140–6.

27. Harirchi I, Arvin A, Vash JH, et al. Frostbite: incidence and predisposing factors in mountaineers. Br J Sports Med 2005;39(12):898–901.

28. Fudge J. Exercise in the Cold: Preventing and Managing Hypothermia and Frostbite Injury. Sports Health 2016;8(2):133.

29. Kempainen RR, Brunette DD. The Evaluation and Management of Accidental Hypothermia. Respir Care 2004;49(2).

30. Duong H, Patel G. Hypothermia. Encyclopedia of the Neurological Sciences 2022;657–8.

31. Danzl DF, Pozos RS. Accidental Hypothermia. N Engl J Med 1994;113(20): 2579–82.

32. Cappaert TA, Stone JA, Castellani JW, et al. National Athletic Trainers' Association Position Statement: Environmental Cold Injuries. J Athl Train 2008;43(6):640.

33. Murphy Jv, Banwell PE, Roberts AHN, et al. Frostbite: pathogenesis and treatment. J Trauma 2000;48(1):171–8.

34. Snell PG, Stray-Gundersen J, Levine BD, et al. American College of Sports Medicine position stand: prevention of cold injuries during exercise. Med Sci Sports Exerc 2006;38(11):103–7.

35. Mistry K, Ondhia C, Levell NJ. A review of trench foot: a disease of the past in the present. Clin Exp Dermatol 2020;45(1):10–4.

36. Cappaert TA, Stone JA, Castellani JW, et al. National Athletic Trainers' Association Position Statement: Environmental Cold Injuries. Available at: http://meridian.allenpress.com/jat/article-pdf/43/6/640/1454631/1062-6050-43_6_640.pdf. Accessed July 12, 2022.

37. davis. MEDICAL ASPECTS OF HARSH ENVIRONMENTS Volume 1.

38. Snell PG, Stray-Gundersen J, Levine BD, et al. American College of Sports Medicine position stand: prevention of cold injuries during exercise. Med Sci Sports Exerc 2006;38(11):103–7.

39. Heil K, Thomas R, Robertson G, et al. Freezing and non-freezing cold weather injuries: a systematic review. Br Med Bull 2016;117(1):79–93.

40. Zafren K. Nonfreezing Cold Injury (Trench Foot). Int J Environ Res Publ Health 2021. https://doi.org/10.3390/ijerph181910482.

41. Glennie JS, Milner R. Non-freezing cold injury. J Roy Nav Med Serv 2014;100(3): 268–71.

42. Cappel JA, Wetter DA. Clinical characteristics, etiologic associations, laboratory findings, treatment, and proposal of diagnostic criteria of pernio (chilblains) in a series of 104 patients at Mayo Clinic, 2000 to 2011. Mayo Clin Proc 2014;89(2): 207–15.

43. Hedrich CM, Fiebig B, Hauck FH, et al. Chilblain lupus erythematosus-a review of literature. Clin Rheumatol 2008. https://doi.org/10.1007/s10067-008-0942-9.

44. Pratt M, Mahmood F, Kirchhof MG. Pharmacologic Treatment of Idiopathic Chilblains (Pernio): A Systematic Review. J Cutan Med Surg 2021;25.

45. RUSTIN MHA, NEWTON JA, SMITH NP, et al. The treatment of chilblains with nifedipine: the results of a pilot study, a double-blind placebo-controlled randomized study and a long-term open trial. Br J Dermatol 1989;120(2):267–75.

46. Prakash S, Weisman MH. Idiopathic chilblains. Am J Med 2009;122(12):1152–5.

47. Recognizing and treating common cold-induced injury in outdo: Medicine & Science in Sports & Exercise. Available at: https://journals.lww.com/acsm-msse/Fulltext/1999/10000/Recognizing_and_treating_common_cold_induced.2.aspx. Accessed July 25, 2022.

48. Healy JD. Excess winter mortality in Europe: a cross country analysis identifying key risk factors. J Epidemiol Community Health 2003;57:784–9. Available at: www.jech.com. Accessed September 6, 2022.

49. Sallis R, Chassay CM. Recognizing and treating common cold-induced injury in outdoor sports. Med Sci Sports Exerc 1999;31(10):1367–73.

50. Wang Y, Saad E, Bonife T, et al. Frostbite Arthritis. Am J Phys Med Rehabil 2016;95(2):e28.

51. Carrera GF, Kozin F, Mccarty DJ. Arthritis after frostbite injury in children. Arthritis Rheum 1979;22(10):1082–7.

52. How Dangerous is Lightning? Available at: https://www.weather.gov/safety/lightning-odds. Accessed May 16, 2022.

53. Scarneo-Miller SE, Walsh Flanagan K, Belval LN, et al. Environmental Concerns Adoption of Lightning Safety Best-Practices Policies in the Secondary School Setting. J Athl Train 2021;56(5):491–8.

54. Jensenius JS. A Detailed Analysis of Lightning Deaths in the United States from 2006 through 2019. 2020.

55. O'Keefe Gatewood M, Zane RD. Lightning Injuries. Emerg Med Clin 2022;22(2):369–403.

56. NWS JetStream - Thunderstorm Hazards: Flash Floods. Available at: https://www.weather.gov/jetstream/flood. Accessed July 4, 2022.

57. NWS Preliminary US Flood Fatality Statistics. Available at: https://www.weather.gov/arx/usflood. Accessed July 4, 2022.

58. NWS JetStream - Thunderstorm Hazards: Flash Floods. Available at: https://www.weather.gov/jetstream/flood. Accessed July 4, 2022.

59. Kentucky woman dies, caught in flash flood in Arizona canyon. Available at: https://www.fox10phoenix.com/news/kentucky-woman-dies-caught-in-flash-flood-in-arizona-canyon1. Accessed July 4, 2022.

60. Flash flooding: a lesser known, but leading weather killer - The Washington Post. Available at: https://www.washingtonpost.com/news/capital-weather-gang/wp/2013/07/11/flash-flooding-a-lesser-known-but-leading-weather-killer/. Accessed July 4, 2022.

61. Utah Flash Floods: Zion Park ID's Seven Killed in Canyon. Available at: https://www.nbcnews.com/news/us-news/utah-flash-floods-zion-park-ids-seven-killed-canyon-n429651. Accessed July 4, 2022.

62. The Narrows Safety - Zion National Park (U.S. National Park Service). Available at: https://www.nps.gov/zion/planyourvisit/narrowssafety.htm. Accessed April 26, 2022.

63. Murdoch D. Altitude sickness.; 2009. Available at: www.clinicalevidence.com. Accessed May 2, 2022.

64. Participants in climbing US 2020 | Statista. Available at: https://www.statista.com/statistics/191233/participants-in-climbing-in-the-us-since-2006/. Accessed April 26, 2022.

65. Prince TS, Thurman J, Huebner K. Acute Mountain Sickness. StatPearls 2022. Available at: https://www.ncbi.nlm.nih.gov/books/NBK430716/. Accessed April 26, 2022.

66. Luks AM, Swenson ER, Bärtsch P. Acute high-altitude sickness. Eur Respir Rev 2017;26(143). https://doi.org/10.1183/16000617.0096-2016.

67. Luks AM, Swenson ER, Bärtsch P. Acute high-altitude sickness. Eur Respir Rev 2017;26(143). https://doi.org/10.1183/16000617.0096-2016.

68. Bärtsch P, Swenson ER. Acute High-Altitude Illnesses. N Engl J Med 2013; 368(24):2294–302.

69. Fulco CS, Muza SR, Beidleman BA, et al. Effect of repeated normobaric hypoxia exposures during sleep on acute mountain sickness, exercise performance, and sleep during exposure to terrestrial altitude. Am J Physiol Regul Integr Comp Physiol 2011;300(2).

70. Richalet JP, Larmignat P, Poitrine E, et al. Physiological risk factors for severe high-altitude illness: a prospective cohort study. Am J Respir Crit Care Med 2012;185(2):192–8.

71. World anti-doping code international standard prohibited list 2022. Available at: www.wada-ama.org. Accessed May 5, 2022.

72. Woods P, Alcock J. High-altitude pulmonary edema. Evol Med Public Health 2021;9(1):118.

73. Murdoch DR. Prevention and Treatment of High-altitude Illness in Travelers. Curr Infect Dis Rep 2004;6(1):43–9.

74. Bartsch P, Maggiorini M, Ritter M, et al. Prevention of high-altitude pulmonary edema by nifedipine. N Engl J Med 1991;325(18):1284–9.

75. Jensen JD, Vincent AL. High Altitude Cerebral Edema. StatPearls. Published online July 20, 2021. Available at: https://www.ncbi.nlm.nih.gov/books/NBK430916/. Accessed May 9, 2022.

76. Li Y, Zhang Y, Zhang Y. Research advances in pathogenesis and prophylactic measures of acute high altitude illness. Respir Med 2018;145:145–52.

77. Cauchy E, Chetaille E, Marchand V, et al. Retrospective study of 70 cases of severe frostbite lesions: a proposed new classification scheme. Wilderness Environ Med 2001;12:255.

78. Rathjen NA, David Shahbodaghi S, Brown JA. Hypothermia and Cold Weather Injuries. Am Fam Physician 2019;100(11). Available at: www.aafp.org/afp. Accessed September 6, 2022.

Emergency Facial Injuries in Athletics

Jessica Tsao, MD, MSc[a], Calvin Eric Hwang, MD[b],*

KEYWORDS

• Facial injury • Facial fracture • Lip laceration • Dental avulsion

KEY POINTS

- Acute vision loss in the setting of trauma is a vision-threatening emergency and warrants urgent ophthalmology evaluation.
- Facial fractures are frequently associated with other serious injuries such as airway compromise and intracranial injury.
- Displaced nasal fractures can be reduced in the acute setting if there is no significant swelling and with proper informed consent.
- Lip lacerations involving the vermillion border should be repaired with special care to achieve anatomic alignment.

OCULAR INJURIES

Introduction

Trauma to the eye is the most common noncongenital cause of vision loss/blindness in patients aged younger than 20 years and is one of the most common causes in patients aged between 21 and 45 years.[1] An estimated 500,000 people are blinded annually because of trauma.[2] The large majority (80%) of these injuries occur in men. In athletes, there is particularly high risk of ocular injury in racket and ball sports. Protective eyewear is important in the prevention of many of these injuries.[1]

Patient Evaluation

Focused evaluation of the eye after traumatic injury should only take place once an overall trauma assessment is completed. Sideline evaluation of the eye after trauma should include external inspection, extraocular movements, pupil assessment, visual acuity, and visual field testing. If appropriate equipment and expertise is available, funduscopic examination and intraocular pressure measurement can be performed. It is critical in the examination of ocular injuries to assess for vision-threatening

[a] Department of Medicine, Stanford University School of Medicine, 866 Campus Drive, Stanford, CA 94305, USA; [b] Department of Orthopaedic Surgery, Stanford University School of Medicine, 341 Galvez Street, Lower Level, Stanford, CA 94305, USA
* Corresponding author.
E-mail address: highlndr@stanford.edu

Clin Sports Med 42 (2023) 463–471
https://doi.org/10.1016/j.csm.2023.02.009
0278-5919/23/© 2023 Elsevier Inc. All rights reserved.
sportsmed.theclinics.com

injuries. These include globe rupture, retrobulbar hematoma, traumatic optic neuropathy, and eyelid laceration. The most common presentation of these injuries is acute vision loss.

Globe ruptures can be diagnosed if there is a penetrating injury to the eyeball with a retained foreign body (open globe rupture) or in the presence of high intraocular pressure after blunt trauma (closed globe rupture). Open globe rupture can be diagnosed by the presence of Seidel sign, visualization of leakage of vitreous fluid after applying fluorescein dye to the eyeball (**Fig. 1**), in addition to the globe appearing collapsed.

Retrobulbar hematoma/hemorrhage is akin to compartment syndrome of the eye. A conscious patient will complain of eye pain and may have proptosis, loss of vision, and the presence of an afferent pupillary defect on examination (**Fig. 2**). However, because these injuries frequently occur in concert with other significant head trauma, initial trauma resuscitation should take place before focused evaluation of the eye.

Traumatic optic neuropathy typically presents with immediate severe vision loss because of shearing, stretching, or contusion of the optic nerve because it transits the optic canal. This is most commonly caused by deceleration injuries and blunt trauma seen in motor vehicle collisions, falls, and assaults. In addition to vision loss, patients with traumatic optic neuropathy may have a relative afferent pupillary defect. Computed tomography (CT) and/or MRI imaging can be used to further evaluate the injury as well as rule out other intracranial causes for the patient's symptoms.

Eyelid lacerations can be vision threatening when they lead to an inability of the eyelids to close properly, thus causing drying of the cornea, ulceration, and potential loss of vision. Specific attention should be given to injuries to the medial and upper eyelid because these may involve the lacrimal duct and levator muscle, respectively.

Treatment

Initial treatment should address any issues affecting airway, breathing, circulation, or spinal cord. Once that has been completed, attention can be turned toward vision-threatening injuries. Patients with any of these vision-threatening injuries should be promptly referred to the emergency department with urgent ophthalmology consultation. Individuals with suspected ruptured globes should have a cup or plastic shield placed on their orbital rim to shield the eye without placing direct pressure on the eyeball. These patients will require urgent surgical repair.

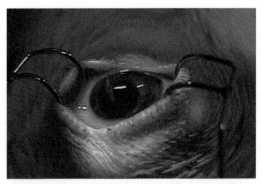

Fig. 1. Seidel lamp. (*From* Mark W. Grinstaff, Designing hydrogel adhesives for corneal wound repair, Biomaterials, Volume 28, Issue 35, 2007, Pages 5205-5214, ISSN 0142-9612, https://doi.org/10.1016/j.biomaterials.2007.08.041. (https://www.sciencedirect.com/science/article/pii/S0142961207007077).)

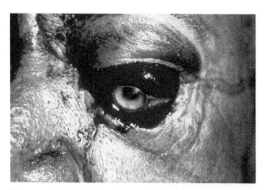

Fig. 2. Retrobulbar hematoma. (*From* Susi Vassallo, Morris Hartstein, David Howard, Jessica Stetz, Traumatic retrobulbar hemorrhage: emergent decompression by lateral canthotomy and cantholysis, The Journal of Emergency Medicine, Volume 22, Issue 3, 2002, Pages 251-256, ISSN 0736-4679, https://doi.org/10.1016/S0736-4679(01)00477-2. (https://www.sciencedirect.com/science/article/pii/S0736467901004772).)

Patients with retrobulbar hematoma ultimately require surgical decompression of the orbit. However, as a temporizing measure, lateral canthotomy and inferior cantholysis can be performed in the emergency department to temporarily relieve intraorbital pressure.

Treatment of traumatic optic neuropathy centers around prompt diagnosis and referral to ophthalmology. Subsequent treatment is controversial as both steroids and/or surgical decompression can be performed.

Simple eyelid lacerations can be cleaned and closed with sutures or glue under local anesthesia. However, more complex lacerations involving the lid margin, lateral or medial canthal regions, medial third of the eyelid, and levator muscle should be addressed by an ophthalmologist due to the sensitive underlying anatomy and functional importance of the injured area. Any laceration resulting in the inability to properly cover the eye should be treated with copious amounts of antibiotic ointment or artificial tears and a wet gauze covering the entire eye to prevent corneal desiccation while awaiting definitive repair.

SUMMARY

Eye injuries are a significant cause of morbidity in sport and prompt recognition of vision-threatening injuries and emergent ophthalmology referral is critical in preventing long-term vision loss.

CLINICS CARE POINTS

- Acute vision loss in the setting of trauma is a vision-threatening emergency and warrants urgent ophthalmology evaluation.
- Patients with suspected globe rupture should have the orbit protected with a cup or plastic shield on the orbital rim to avoid applying direct pressure to the eye.
- Copious amounts of antibiotic ointment or artificial tears and a wet gauze should be used in patients with eyelid lacerations until they can be evaluated by ophthalmology.

NASAL INJURIES
Introduction

Nasal injuries are common in sports because the nose is the most commonly fractured bone in the adult face and epistaxis occurs frequently in the setting of nasal trauma, requiring removal from activity until addressed.[1] The nose is composed of both bony and cartilaginous structures with the 2 nasal bones forming the bridge of the nose to support the underlying cartilaginous structures.[3] Within the nose, there is an extensive network of blood vessels, most notable of which is Kiesselbach plexus located in the anterior nasal septum and is the most common source of bleeding posttrauma.

Patient Evaluation

Although the nose can be part of the initial trauma evaluation (ABCs), focused evaluation of nasal injuries should only occur once that initial evaluation has been completed. Nasal fractures commonly present with epistaxis, an obvious deformity, and tenderness on examination. In patients with more subtle findings, the use of a mirror or front facing phone camera can be helpful for the patient to visually confirm a new deformity. Old photos on the patient's phone or driver's license can also help with the baseline appearance. The diagnosis of an isolated nasal fracture can be made clinically and routine x-rays or CT imaging are not required if there is no significant concern for other underlying injuries.

The presence of clear rhinorrhea or other nonbloody fluid drainage is concerning for a cerebrospinal fluid (CSF) leak because of fracture of the underlying cribriform plate and would warrant CT imaging. Midface fractures commonly occur with nasal fractures and would require referral to plastic or oral maxillofacial surgery (see "Facial fractures" section). Close attention should also be given to the nasal septum for the presence of a septal hematoma. This would present as a purple or blue area of swelling in the nasal septum (**Fig. 3**) and would require drainage to prevent abscess formation, septal perforation, and/or development of a saddle nose deformity.

Treatment

In patients with an isolated displaced nasal fracture, closed reduction can be considered in the acute setting. However, patients should be counseled on the potential need

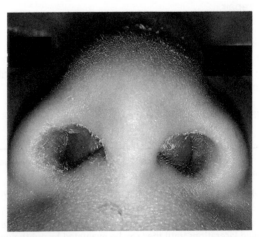

Fig. 3. Septal hematoma. (*From* Chandran, A., Sakthivel, P. & Singh, C.A. A Swollen Nose – Nasal Septal Hematoma. Indian J Pediatr 87, 88 (2020). https://doi.org/10.1007/s12098-019-03052-w.)

for further reduction and/or rhinoplasty based on persistent deformities. This can occur in up to 50% of cases. Patients with a CSF leak will need to be referred to otolaryngology and started on antibiotics due to the risk of meningitis. Septal hematomas should be drained urgently to prevent complications. This can be performed by a sports medicine physician with experience in the procedure or in the local emergency department.

SUMMARY

Nasal injuries are frequently encountered in sport and the sports medicine physician should be well versed in the diagnosis and management of nasal fractures and septal hematomas.

CLINICS CARE POINTS

- Displaced nasal fractures can be reduced in the acute setting if there is no significant swelling and with proper informed consent.
- Clear rhinorrhea in the setting of facial trauma should raise concern for a CSF leak.
- Septal hematomas must be promptly identified and drained to prevent abscess formation, septal perforation, and/or development of saddle nose deformity.

FACIAL FRACTURES
Introduction

Facial fractures are also quite common in sports, with epidemiological studies showing that facial fractures comprise between 4% and 18% of all sports-related injuries.[1] Facial fractures are more common in men than in women.[4] Due to the complexity of the bony facial anatomy, there are a number of different fracture types that can occur, and knowledge of these is crucial for sports physicians to ensure appropriate evaluation and treatment.

Patient Evaluation

With the high-energy trauma required for most facial fractures, airway compromise is a real risk due to soft tissue edema, hemorrhage, and instability. Only when the airway is secured, should a thorough examination of the face including evaluation of the cranial nerves be performed. In general, CT is the gold standard for the diagnosis of facial fractures and will thus require referral to a medical center; however, examination of the athlete can give clues to the potential injury. Further, up to 6% of patients with facial trauma can develop vision loss, making a detailed eye examination to evaluate for ocular injury critical.[5]

Orbital blowout fractures typically occur when a traumatic force applied to the eye is transmitted to the fragile inferior orbit causing a fracture. When evaluating orbital fractures, a thorough examination of the eye is necessary to exclude vision-threatening injuries. Physical examination findings include enophthalmos, infraorbital numbness, and crepitus or pain with palpation of the orbital rim. Extraocular movements should be carefully checked to look for any evidence of ocular muscle entrapment.[5]

The zygoma provides the bony structure for the cheek, and its location on the face leads to frequent injury. Fractures of the zygoma often present with flattening of the cheek; however, other examination findings include tilting appearance of the globe, diplopia, infraorbital numbness, and crepitus as the zygoma makes up a portion of the orbit and maxillary sinus. Trismus can also be seen as the zygoma is an attachment point for the masseter.[1,5]

Midface fractures are generally the result of high-energy trauma and are classified according to fracture patterns originally described by the French surgeon René LeFort in 1901 (**Fig. 4**). These fractures often result in facial instability, identifiable by mobility of the structures of the midface when manipulated on examination. Which structures are mobile depends on the degree of fracture. LeFort I fractures are horizontal fractures through the maxilla, separating the maxilla and hard palate from the rest of the midface, with only the hard palate mobile on examination. LeFort II fractures are pyramidal fractures involving the central maxilla and hard palate. On examination, LeFort II fractures will demonstrate movement of the hard palate and nose. LeFort III fractures involve a complete separation of the midface from the rest of the cranium with fractures through the orbits, nasal bridge, and extending laterally through the zygomatic arch. In LeFort III fractures, the entire midface will be mobile, except for the eyes, which are held in place by the optic nerve.[5]

Athletes with mandibular trauma should be evaluated for dental malocclusion, pain with movement of the jaw, and numbness of the lower lip (inferior alveolar nerve injury), which are all common presenting symptoms for mandible fracture. The majority of mandibular fractures are bilateral due to the ring-like nature of the mandible. If a mandible fracture is suspected, close inspection of the oropharynx is warranted to identify any dental trauma as well as small breaks in the oral mucosa, which indicate an open fracture.

Treatment

All open fractures should receive prophylactic antibiotics and generally require admission for operative repair. For closed fractures, treatment depends on the location and the degree of displacement. Orbital fractures should receive prophylactic antibiotics to cover sinus pathogens, nose-blowing precautions, and specialist evaluation because there is some controversy regarding timing of repair. Nondisplaced zygoma fractures can be managed nonoperatively; however, surgical repair of all displaced and comminuted zygoma fractures is required and should be performed within 2 weeks to prevent facial deformity.[1] Additionally, fractures with evidence of entrapment should receive

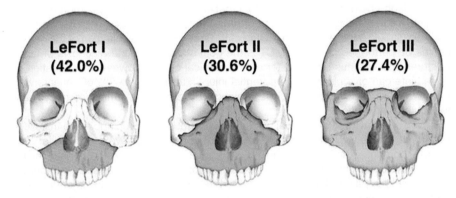

Fig. 4. Le Fort classification. (*From* Kevin C. Lee, Sung-Kiang Chuang, Sidney B. Eisig, The Characteristics and Cost of Le Fort Fractures: A Review of 519 Cases From a Nationwide Sample, Journal of Oral and Maxillofacial Surgery, Volume 77, Issue 6, 2019, Pages 1218-1226, ISSN 0278-2391, https://doi.org/10.1016/j.joms.2019.01.060. (https://www.sciencedirect.com/science/article/pii/S0278239119301363).)

emergent specialist referral. LeFort fractures also require admission to manage associated injuries, IV antibiotics, and surgical repair, and all athletes with suspected midface fractures should be evaluated in the emergency department. Closed mandible fractures can be managed initially with a Barton bandage to stabilize the fracture and reduce pain, and these patients can be given urgent out-patient follow-up.[5]

SUMMARY

Facial fractures constitute a significant portion of all sports-related injuries, and sports physicians should be aware of the different types of fractures and their treatment. These are often high-energy injuries and care should be taken to evaluate for airway compromise and hemodynamic instability. Most athletes with suspected facial fractures will require evaluation at a medical facility to determine the extent of the injury.

CLINICS CARE POINTS

- Facial fractures are frequently associated with other serious injuries such as airway compromise and intracranial injury.
- CT is the gold standard for diagnosis of most facial fractures, and all patients with suspected facial fractures except isolated nasal bone fractures should get advanced imaging to confirm the diagnosis and for prognostication.
- All open fractures should be admitted for IV antibiotics and surgical repair.

DENTAL AND ORAL TRAUMA
Introduction

Sports-related injury accounts for an estimated 4% to 39% of dental trauma and is the most common cause of dental trauma in adolescents.[6,7] Although the use of mouth protection (mouthguards, facemasks, and so forth) has been shown to reduce the risk for oral trauma, it still remains a significant source of morbidity with an estimated cost of up to US$15,000 per injured tooth.[6] Due to the unique and sometimes complex nature of these injuries, it is imperative that physicians doing sideline coverage are familiar with how to evaluate and treat dental and oral injuries.

Patient Evaluation

As with other facial injuries, athletes with dental and oral trauma should first be evaluated for evidence of airway compromise and hemodynamic instability. Any evidence of these should prompt immediate referral to the hospital. The athlete should also be evaluated for concussion and other head and neck injuries. Those with isolated dental and oral trauma can often be treated by the sports physician with urgent referral to a dentist.

Normal tooth anatomy consists of a layer of hard enamel, which covers the dentin, itself covering the pulp, which is the tooth's neurovascular supply. Teeth should be carefully examined for fracture or luxation. Tooth fractures are categorized using the Ellis classification according to which structures are involved and are typically easily identifiable on examination (**Fig. 5**). Ellis I fractures are isolated enamel fractures. Ellis II fractures result in exposed dentin, which is distinguishable by a yellow hue different from the enamel. In Ellis III fractures, there is exposure of the tooth pulp, which is identified by bleeding or exposed pink-red tissue in the tooth on examination.[8] Care should also be taken to evaluate for fractures of the alveolar ridge, which often occur concomitantly with other dental trauma.

The presence of a dental injury should prompt evaluation for oral lacerations because these often occur concurrently. Oral lacerations require particular attention for the involvement of the vermilion border of the lip as well as the depth of the laceration as vermillion border injuries and through-and-through lacerations require different management. All lacerations should be evaluated for hemostasis, which can typically be achieved with direct pressure.

Treatment

Treatment of dental fractures is based on the Ellis classification. Isolated enamel fractures (Ellis I) do not require any immediate treatment. Ellis II and Ellis III fractures are usually air sensitive and use of a dental wax or a thin layer of a calcium hydroxide base followed by dental cement can protect the tooth from further damage and provide pain relief until the athlete is able to see a dentist. Alveolar ridge fractures require flexible fixation placed by a dentist or oral surgeon for stabilization. Ellis Class I injuries do not require urgent dental referral, whereas Ellis II, Ellis III, and alveolar fractures should have an urgent dental referral.[1,8]

For tooth avulsions, on-field treatment involves gently removing any debris with sterile saline before placing the tooth back into the socket. The avulsed tooth should be handled only by the crown to prevent damage to the root. Teeth, which are reimplanted within 30 minutes, have a greater than 90% chance of survival.[1] These injuries require immediate evaluation by a dentist. An exception to this is avulsed primary teeth, which should not be reimplanted. Athletes with avulsed teeth should have their tetanus updated, if necessary, and given antibiotic prophylaxis with doxycycline.[8]

Lip lacerations can be repaired primarily; however, special attention should be paid to align the vermillion border as closely as possible to achieve a good cosmetic outcome. Isolated lacerations of the oral mucosa, which approximate well and do not gape open do not require repair. Through-and-through lacerations should be repaired in layers with absorbable sutures used to first close the mucosal layer, followed by the orbis orbicularis fascia, and finally the skin.[9] The use of nerve blocks

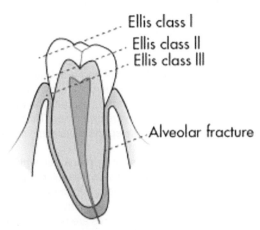

Fig. 5. Ellis classification. (*From* Leathers RD, Gowans RE. Management of alveolar and dental fractures. In: Miloro M, editor. Peterson's principles of oral and maxillofacial surgery. 2nd ed. Hamilton: BC Decker; 2004. (A) p.388; (B) p.389; (C) p.390; (D) p.387.)

rather than local infiltration of anesthetic is helpful to maintain the normal anatomy allowing for better visualization of the alignment.

SUMMARY

Dental and oral injuries are a common occurrence in sport. Initial evaluation should always begin with an assessment of the patient's airway, breathing, circulation, as well as identification of associated injuries. Tooth avulsions are the only true dental emergency. Oral lacerations frequently do not require repair; however, special attention should be paid to lip lacerations involving the vermillion border. Most tooth and oral lacerations can be treated on the field with urgent referral to a dentist.

CLINICS CARE POINTS

- Always ensure that the airway is intact before further evaluation of dental and oral trauma.
- Avulsed teeth should be placed back into the socket as soon as possible with prompt dental follow-up.
- Lip lacerations involving the vermillion border should be repaired with special care to achieve anatomic alignment.

DISCLOSURE

The authors declare no commercial or financial conflicts of interest or any outside funding sources.

REFERENCES

1. Reehal P. Facial injury in sport. Curr Sports Med Rep 2010;9(1):27–34.
2. Perry M, Dancey A, Mireskandari K, et al. Emergency care in facial trauma–a maxillofacial and ophthalmic perspective. Injury 2005;36(8):875–96.
3. Patel Y, Goljan P, Pierce TP, et al. Management of nasal fractures in sports. Sports Med 2017;47(10):1919–23.
4. Romeo SJ, Hawley CJ, Romeo MW, et al. Sideline management of facial injuries. Curr Sports Med Rep 2007;6(3):155–61.
5. Hedayati T, Amin DP. Trauma to the face, Chapter: 259. In: Tintinalli's emergency medicine: a comprehensive study guide, 9e. USA: McGraw-Hill Education; 2020.
6. Gould T.E., Jesunathadas M., Nazarenko S., et al., Chapter 6-mouth protection in sports, In: Subic A., *Materials in sports equipment*, 2nd Edition, 2019, Woodhead Publishing, Sawston, UK, 199–231, Woodhead publishing series in composites science and engineering.
7. Lam R. Epidemiology and outcomes of traumatic dental injuries: a review of the literature. Aust Dent J 2016;1(61 Suppl):4–20.
8. Beaudreau RW. Oral and dental emergencies, Chapter: 245. In: *Tintinalli's emergency medicine: a comprehensive study guide, 9e*. USA: McGraw-Hill Education; 2020.
9. Coates WC. Face and scalp lacerations, Chapter: 42. In: *Tintinalli's emergency medicine: a comprehensive study guide, 9e*. USA: McGraw-Hill Education; 2020.

Head Injuries and Emergencies in Sports

Ashwin L. Rao, MD[a,b,*], Leina'ala Song, MD[b,c], Georgia Griffin, MD[b,d]

KEYWORDS

- Head injury • Concussion • Fracture • Laceration

KEY POINTS

- Head injuries represent an important injury designation, for which sports medicine providers should be prepared to recognize, manage, and appropriately triage.
- Concussions represent a form of mild traumatic brain injury, with both physiologic and short-term clinical impacts, and require careful management before return to play.
- On-field evaluation of head injuries requires a stepwise process for evaluating airway, breathing, circulation, disability, and trauma (ABCDE).
- Standardized evaluation tools for concussion are important in assessing readiness for return to play.

INTRODUCTION
Definition of Head Injury

The term "head injury" refers to damage caused by external forces, blows, or head trauma brought on by acceleration and deceleration **Box 1**. Specifically, it is a clinically identifiable injury that is distinct from traumatic brain injury (TBI) which denotes damage to the brain itself. Injuries can be direct or indirect. Direct trauma results in damage to the skull and brain-dependent upon factors such as velocity, direction, force magnitude, surface area, and mass of the striking object, as well as vasogenic and elastic properties of the underlying brain tissue. Indirect trauma occurs without direct mechanical impact, but with acceleration, deceleration, pressure waves, and/or shearing forces that cause intracranial disruption and insult as the brain strikes the skull or dura (such as contrecoup contusion) or injury to bridging subdural vessels.

[a] Department of Family Medicine, Section of Sports Medicine, University of Washington, Seattle, WA, USA; [b] University of Washington Sports Medicine Center, 3800 Montlake Boulevard NE, Box 354060, Seattle, WA 98195, USA; [c] Department of Family Medicine, Section of Sports Medicine, University of Washington, Seattle, WA, USA; [d] Department of Family Medicine, Section of Sports Medicine, University of Washington, Seattle Children's Hospital, Seattle, WA, USA
* Corresponding author.
E-mail address: ashwin@uw.edu

Clin Sports Med 42 (2023) 473–489
https://doi.org/10.1016/j.csm.2023.02.010
0278-5919/23/Published by Elsevier Inc.

Box 1
Glasgow coma scale scoring

Eye-Opening Response (Maximum score of 4)
- Spontaneously (4)
- To voice (3)
- To pain (3)
- No response (1)

Verbal Response (Maximum score of 5)
- Oriented to time, place, person (5)
- Confused (4)
- Inappropriate words (3)
- Incomprehensible sounds (2)
- No response (1)

Motor Response (Maximum score of 6)
- Obeys commands (6)
- Localizes pain (5)
- Withdrawal from pain (4)
- Abnormal flexion (decorticate) (3)
- Abnormal extension (decerebrate) (2)
- No response (1)

Brain injuries may be classified by severity, with subsequent temporary or permanent symptoms. Although the large majority of outcomes are mild, brain injury can result in permanent disability or death. In sports, moderate and severe brain injuries usually occur with high velocity or contact and collision sports.

Cerebral injury can induce brain surface bruising and parenchymal damage, including damage to the parenchymal blood vessels, with subsequent edema and petechial hemorrhage. Secondary insults following brain injury such as hypoxia or hypotension, cause a cascade of cytotoxic events including inflammatory response, free radical production, neurotransmitter dysregulation, and metabolic imbalance.

TYPES OF HEAD INJURIES
Concussion

Concussion is defined as a transient impairment of brain function induced by a force transmitted to the head. Concussion is a subset of mild TBI.[1] The signs and symptoms of acute concussion typically fall into four categories: physical (eg, headache, sensitivity to noise or light, dizziness, balance problems, blurry vision, drowsiness, nausea, and vomiting), cognitive (eg, confusion, difficulty concentrating, feeling slowed down, and difficulty remembering new information), emotional (eg, irritability, sadness, feeling more emotional, nervousness or anxiety), and sleep (eg, sleeping more than usual, sleeping less than usual, and trouble falling asleep).[2] The clinical signs and symptoms of concussion cannot be explained by other etiologies, such as drug, alcohol, or medication use, mental illness, or other injuries (such as cervical injuries or peripheral vestibular dysfunction) or other comorbidities (such psychological factors or coexisting medical conditions).[1]

Concussion symptoms are mediated by a complex cascade of ionic, metabolic, and pathophysiologic events. The current understanding is that stress applied to neurons leads to changes in intracellular ion concentrations, the indiscriminate release of neurotransmitters, mitochondrial dysfunction leading to the production of reactive oxygen species, and increased glucose utilization to restore ion imbalances. Meanwhile, injury-associated decreased resting cerebral blood flow (CBF) generates an energy mismatch.[3-8] The degree of brain injury depends on the initial impact severity, secondary insults, as well as underlying genetic and molecular response.

Scalp Laceration

Scalp lacerations may occur through blunt force trauma or contact with a sharp object. The severity of this injury can be correlated to scalp soft tissue anatomy, specifically loose areolar attachments. The loose areolar connective tissue serves as the attachment between the epicranial aponeurosis and pericranium layers of the scalp, but also a potential space for fluid collection. Loose areolar attachments can cause large subgaleal hematomas as blood easily "dissects" through the tissue. Careful history and exam should be done to assess for the mechanism of injury, foreign bodies, tetanus status, risk or evidence of infection, and for factors that could inhibit wound healing such as immunocompromised state, diabetes mellitus, steroid, or substance use. Small foreign bodies should be removed promptly and minimize risk of exposure, however penetrating intracranial foreign bodies should not be removed so as not to worsen bleeding. Achieving hemostasis is critical though can be difficult, as large blood vessels of the scalp often do not constrict completely when lacerated. On the sidelines, proper use of equipment should be emphasized to minimize risk complications from laceration. Players can generally return to play if hemostasis is achieved and an adequate dressing can be applied without restrictions.

Skull Fracture

Skull fractures involve a break or compromise to the calvarium, typically occurring through application of a substantial, externally applied force that compromises the integrity of the bones constituting the cranium. Fracture characteristic depends on impact location and force, resulting in depressed, basilar, extra-axial (within the skull but outside the brain tissue), or intra-axial (within brain tissue itself) injuries. When suspected, a non-contrast head computed tomography (CT) scan with bone windows is the diagnostic standard.

Linear fractures are singular and go through the entire skull thickness. They are usually secondary to low-energy blunt trauma. Although most are not clinically significant, if they cross the middle meningeal groove or major dural sinuses, they can cause epidural hematomas or sutural diastasis if they extend into the suture line.

Depressed fractures typically occur over parietal or temporal areas due to direct impact with blunt objects. These are at higher risk for significant brain injury and complications.

Basilar skull fractures must be paid special attention as they have proximity to the middle cerebral artery and hematomas can compress and entrap cranial nerves that pass through the basal foramina, otic canal or cavernous sinuses, and the facial nerve.

Epidural Hematoma

Epidural hematomas are extra-axial intracranial lesions, related to the compromise of blood vessels between the skull and dura. They are most frequently a consequence of a direct impact temporoparietal injury causing fracture across the middle meningeal artery, vein, or dural sinus. Hematoma formation occurs as the dura is dissected away from the skull. Non-contrast CT will show a biconvex lenticular lesion that does not extend beyond dural attachments.

The classic presentation is a direct head trauma with an initial brief level of decreased consciousness, followed by a lucid interval where the patient's level of consciousness is near baseline, then a second episode of significantly decreased consciousness. Care must be taken to ensure early recognition which significantly improves outcomes.

Subdural Hematoma

Subdural hematomas are also extra-axial intracranial lesions. They are more common than epidural hematomas and occur between the dura and the brain, usually in adults with brain atrophy. Non-contrast CT will show a lesion that extends beyond suture lines and follows the contour of the tentorium.

Older patients or alcoholics with brain atrophy have bridging vessels that have to traverse farther distances and are vulnerable to rupture with acceleration-deceleration forces. Expanding hematoma on the underlying tissue develops slowly as the venous blood accumulates, but causes prolonged pressure and can result in significant tissue damage. Patients must be monitored for developing neurologic dysfunction and risk of acute herniation syndrome.

Subarachnoid Hemorrhage

Traumatic subarachnoid hemorrhage, another extra-axial intracranial lesion, is associated with high morbidity and mortality. Tears of the small subarachnoid vessels can cause subarachnoid hemorrhage within the cerebrospinal fluid (CSF) and meningeal intima. Non-contrast CT will show increased density within the basilar cisterns, interhemispheric fissures, and sulci. Presenting Glasgow Coma Scale (GCS) and outcome are correlated with the amount of blood within the hemorrhage. Those associated with GCS abnormalities require intervention.

Intracerebral Hemorrhage

Intracerebral hemorrhage refers to the condition where a hematoma forms within the brain parenchyma and sometimes extends into the ventricles. Shearing forces that stretch the smaller arterioles over the cranial vault cause tearing and small petechial hemorrhages that cause deep intracerebral hemorrhages. The most common presentation is a sudden onset of focal neurological deficits.

A small number of these are non-traumatic, with uncontrolled chronic hypertension, amyloid angiography, vascular malformations, neoplasms, and use of anticoagulants or drug use being important risk factors. Traumatic intracranial hemorrhage has been shown to tend toward expanding over time. Intracerebral hematoma may not be seen on CT until several hours after the injury and become further demarcated with time. If lesions degrade a few days after the initial injury, findings may instead represent cerebral contusion. Most intracerebral hematomas are multiple and occur in fronto-temporal lobes. In contrast, traumatic intracerebellar hematomas occur with direct occipital blows.

Diffuse Axonal Injury

Diffuse axonal injury, also known as traumatic axonal injury, occurs after blunt trauma to the brain. White matter injury occurs from acceleration and deceleration shearing forces. The axonal stretching that occurs causes a cascade of axolemmal disruption, neurofilament compaction, microtubule disassembly, and ion flux, causing axonal swelling and disconnection, ultimately leading to axonal death. Neuronal degeneration can continue to occur up to months after the trauma. Gross damage is seen at the gray and white matter junction. This predilection occurs because of differing relative mass per volume of the gray and white matter which are particularly vulnerable in these shearing injuries.

Diffuse axonal injury is largely a clinical diagnosis, as radiographic findings are often non-specific. Lesions can be seen at the gray–white matter junction, most often in the corpus callosum or brainstem. CT of the head may show small punctate hemorrhages of the white matter tracts, but MRI is the modality of choice. Specifically, diffuse tensor imaging is a better diagnostic imaging modality.

HEAD INJURY COMPLICATIONS
Secondary Brain Injury

Secondary brain injury is a cellular injury that occurs after a primary brain injury (laceration, contusion, hemorrhage), set off by a cascade of secondary local and systemic events. Hypoxia, hypotension, hypertension, brain ischemia, increased intracranial pressure (ICP), anemia, hyperpyrexia, and hypoglycemia all mediate secondary brain injury and are important to prevent and treat following TBI.

Although some inflammation may facilitate repair following injury, maladaptive inflammation may promote secondary injury. Numerous observational studies describe an association between elevated proinflammatory cytokines and neurologic outcome and mortality, however, the point at which inflammation becomes pathologic remains unknown.[9]

Brain injury causes increased CBF, vascular dilation, and disruption of the blood–brain barrier. This leads to dysregulation of extracellular ion and neurotransmitter concentrations and resulting vasogenic edema. This cascade leads to increased ICP. Cerebral perfusion pressure (CPP) is defined as the difference between mean arterial pressure (MAP) and ICP and represents the resistance of CBF reaching the brain. This is expressed as the equation: $CCP = MAP\text{–}ICP$.

A steady rate of CBF, in spite of changes in arterial pressure, is maintained through a process called autoregulation. Autoregulation is disrupted at a CPP of <40 mm Hg, which can occur in the setting of elevated ICP or decreased MAP. Injured cerebral blood vessels may also lose the ability to regulate CBF. Hypercarbia exacerbates cerebral arterial dilation, contributing to increased ICP. The brain is also very dependent on oxygen, thus, short periods of hypoxia can have detrimental effects on brain function. Hyperpyrexia (core body temperature >38.5°C) is thought to increase proinflammatory cytokines and blood flow, also contributing to increased ICP.[10,11] Hypotension causes a fall in CCP.

Second-Impact Syndrome

Second-impact syndrome is an exceptionally rare, potentially fatal consequence of repeated mild TBI before symptoms from the first head trauma have resolved, resulting in diffuse brain swelling.[12] It primarily affects children and young adults, thus, making it imperative to identify a first concussion in youth athletes and avoiding impact sports participation before full resolution of concussion signs and symptoms. The pathophysiology and risk factors are controversial and more research is needed.[13,14]

Post-Traumatic Seizure

Convulsions after a TBI can be classified based on their temporal relationship to the injury. Post-traumatic seizures are commonly divided into three categories: (1) impact (within seconds), (2) early (within 7 days), or (3) late (greater than 7 days).[15] Impact seizures are also called concussive convulsions, and are thought to be non-epileptic and benign. Conversely, late seizures implicate structural brain damage and can turn into post-traumatic epilepsy (PTE).[16] Mild TBIs have minuscule risk of PTE, however, the risk increases with TBI severity, cortical contusion, epidural or subdural hematoma, intracerebral hemorrhage, and depressed skull fracture. Seizures also can cause hypoxia, hypercarbia, and increased ICP, furthering brain injury.

Chronic Traumatic Brain Injury

Repeated head trauma has been associated with early dementia, changes in cognition, movement, and more recently with mood, personality, and behavior, albeit with controversy. Chronic traumatic encephalopathy (CTE) refers to a wide array of neurodegenerative changes identified in neuropathology, including tau and amyloid-beta deposits, brain atrophy, axonal degeneration, and persistent neuroinflammation. Neuropathologic changes such as brain atrophy have also been noted after a single TBI. It is unknown what dose of head trauma (ie, what cumulative combination of sub-concussive head blows and TBI) triggers neurodegeneration. The clinical criteria and epidemiology of CTE remains poorly defined and further research is needed[17]

ON-FIELD EVALUATION OF HEAD INJURIES
ABCDE

Evaluation of traumatic head injury begins with an expedited primary survey beginning with assessing airway, breathing, and circulation with hemorrhage control ("ABCs"). The secondary survey to evaluate for disability ("D") including brain injury and neurologic compromise, as well as evidence of external signs of trauma ("E") should take place once the athlete has been safely removed from the field.

It is imperative to prevent and correct reversible conditions that can alter the mental status and worsen neurologic function, including hypoxia, hypotension, hypoglycemia, anemia, and hyperpyrexia. It is important to monitor head-injured athletes' breathing. Hypoxia leads to increased morbidity and mortality and must be avoided. Although out-of-hospital endotracheal intubation is a topic of controversy, if the airway is compromised or unable to keep oxygen saturation above 90% with supplemental oxygen, definitive airway management should be considered and only deferred if transport time is short. It is also crucial to monitor and manage blood pressure, particularly if there is evidence of blood loss or hemorrhage. Systolic blood pressure should be kept above 90 mm Hg.

Red Flags

- Clinical findings suggestive of basilar skull fractures such as blood in the ear canal, hemotympanum, rhinorrhea, otorrhea, retroauricular hematoma (Battle's sign), periorbital ecchymosis (raccoon sign), cranial nerve deficits, facial paralysis, decreased auditory acuity, tinnitus, nystagmus, or dizziness.
- CSF may leak from the nose or ear when there is a fracture of the cranium with disruption of the dura.
- Signs of cervical spine injury (eg, cervical fracture, carotid artery dissection, and spinal cord injury) include midline cervical tenderness and painful cervical range of motion. If gentle cervical range of motion is met with pain or resistance, range of motion testing should be stopped.

Reasons for immediate removal from practice or competition include signs of concussion, loss of consciousness (LOC), impact seizure, tonic posturing, gross motor instability, confusion, or amnesia.[3]

Glasgow Coma Scale

The GCS is an objective measurement of the level of consciousness.[18,19] It assesses three aspects of responsiveness: eye-opening, verbal, and motor, using a scale ranging from 3 at the worst to 15 at the best (**Box 2**). The strongest outcome predictor is the motor response.[20–22] GCS is used to categorize TBI into mild (GCS 13–15), moderate (GCS 9–12), and severe (GCS 3–8) categories. Serial GCS evaluations are also helpful for monitoring neurologic function, and declining GCS may portend an expanding intracranial hematoma.

Although GCS is nearly universally used and enables reliable and rapid neurologic assessment, it has limitations. Periorbital or ocular trauma or edema may affect eye response evaluation. Mandibular trauma or edema may affect verbal response. The spinal cord, plexus, or peripheral nerve injury may affect motor response. A full cranial nerve assessment should also be done when feasible.

A pupillary exam should be performed on anyone with a head injury. The examiner should assess for pupil shape, size, response to light, and eye movement, including accommodation. It is important for clinicians to know that up to one-fifth of normal individuals have anisocoria,[23] though both pupils should react to light equally. In a fully conscious athlete who has sustained a blow near the eye, a dilated fixed pupil is more likely due to trauma to the short ciliary nerves as opposed to brain herniation causing compression of the third cranial nerve. Mid-sized non-reactive bilateral pupils suggest midbrain damage, and dilated non-reactive bilateral pupils is a sign of anoxia and ischemia to the brain.[24] Concussions frequently lead to abnormalities in eye tracking.

Cervical Spine

Cervical spine injury (CSI) is common in sports, with football and ice hockey being the sports shown to be at the highest risk. When a CSI is suspected, it is essential to have a well-rehearsed Emergency Action Plan (EAP) because optimizing pre-hospital care can mitigate poor outcomes. Pre-hospital EAPs should be developed preemptively using evidence-based guidelines adapted as best as possible to team resources and location conditions. Scenario-based and venue-specific training should be done at least annually with all members of the interdisciplinary team. In 2020, the National Athletic Trainer's Association published consensus recommendations on the

---

Box 2
Key elements of the secondary survey in head injuries

1. Inspection: Examine the scalp, skull, and face for cranial fractures, deformities, binocular hematomas, and Battle sign. An otoscope may be used to look for CSF and/or blood leakage from the ears, mouth, and nose.

2. Palpation: Palpate gently for Indentations or depressed skull fractures. Assess for neck tenderness.

3. Neurologic assessment: Determine GCS. Examine the pupils for size, equality, and light reflex. Evaluate balance and coordination. Assess for any neck pain.

4. Focused history:
   1. Ask the athlete to recall events surrounding the incident
   2. Amnesia before and after the incident and for how long
   3. Ask about clinically significant symptoms such as severe headache, nausea, paresthesias, weakness, and visual defects.
   4. Inquire about a sweet taste in the mouth, which may be due to CSF leakage.
   5. Medical history such as coagulopathies, use of anticoagulants or antiplatelets
   6. Allergies
   7. Medications
   8. Family history of stroke, subarachnoid bleeding, bleeding disorders

pre-hospital care of the injured athlete with a suspected catastrophic CSI which have been summarized here.

When an injured athlete has a suspected CSI, rapid and safe transportation to a Level I or II trauma center should be prioritized, as these centers are best equipped to manage such injuries. Before transport, airway safety should be assessed and access established before transport. Any facemasks should be removed, which will be discussed further in the next section.

Methods of transfer and spinal-motion restriction have been studied to find which are associated with best outcomes for athletes with suspected CSI. When turning a prone athlete, the log-roll-push techniques have been shown to be superior to log-roll-pull techniques. In supine athletes, the 8-person lift-and-slide has been shown to cause less spinal movement than the log-roll. Therefore for suspected CSIs, whenever possible, the 8-person lift-and-slide technique should be used for supine athletes and a log-roll-push technique for prone athletes.

Helmet and Facemask Removal

For sports utilizing headgear, face masks should be removed to ensure airway access before transfer to the designated trauma center when a CSI is suspected. Proper equipment should be used by trained personnel to do so with minimal cervical spine motion, as the highest priority is maintaining alignment of the cervical spine. Ideally one trained on-site medical personnel would be maintaining cervical stabilization whereas another removes the facemask.

Maintenance of circulation, airway, and breathing is the highest priority, and if compromised, helmet and shoulder pads should be removed. When deciding whether to remove the helmet and shoulder pads in a stable athlete, providers should consider athlete weight, sport, available immobilization devices, and equipment make and model. If helmet removal is attempted without shoulder pad removal, studies have shown there is a small but statistically significant amount of cervical movement that occurs portending risk of cervical spine malalignment. There has been no evidence of statistically significant differences in the alignment of the cervical spine when the helmet and shoulder pads are removed versus when they are left on. Therefore, it is left to the discretion of the responding personnel, and the chosen protocol should be well-rehearsed in their EAP.

OFF-FIELD EVALUATION OF HEAD INJURIES

The player with head injury should be immediately removed from play and brought to the sideline where the primary survey should be repeated. Then a secondary survey including head-to-toe assessment should be conducted (see **Box 2**).

If the athlete is alert, responsive, stable, pain-free, and able to stand and walk unassisted, the next step in assessment is a sideline concussion evaluation. Concussion assessment should take place in a distraction-free environment. If concussion is suspected but not confirmed, then the athlete should be removed from play and serial evaluations are recommended.[3] If a CSI is suspected, the patient should be immobilized on a spine board and transported by emergency medical personnel to a leve1 or 2 trauma center for further evaluation.

Standardized Assessment Tools

Sideline assessment tools have several limitations including low test-retest reliability as well as low sensitivity and specificity.[3] It is important to know an athlete's baseline function on these assessments. Symptoms remain the most sensitive indicator of a concussion.[25,26]

The Concussion in Sport Group recommends the SCAT5 and the Child SCAT5 for assessing a suspected concussion. The SCAT5 consists of a brief neurologic examination, a symptom checklist, a brief cognitive assessment (SAC), and a balance assessment (BESS). The goal of these tools is to aid in clinical assessment of concussion. Diagnosis of concussion necessitates a clear mechanism consistent with concussion, characteristic signs, symptoms, and time course of concussion, and no other cause explaining the observed findings.[3] If the athlete is deemed unlikely to have sustained a concussion, then continued participation should be safe. If the athlete is diagnosed with a concussion or probable concussion, then they should be removed from participation with no same-day return to play.[3]

Other Testing: Vestibular/Ocular Motor Screening and King-Devick Test

Vestibular symptoms occur in 67% to 77% and ocular impairment occurs in 45% of sports-related concussions.[27,28] The Vestibular/Ocular Motor Screening (VOMS) tool evaluates the following domains: smooth pursuits (ability to follow slowly moving target vertically and horizontally); convergence distance (ability to view a near target without double vision, with <6 cm from nose considered normal); saccades (ability for eyes to move quickly between targets); the vestibular ocular reflex (ability to stabilize vision as the head moves); vestibular motion sensitivity (ability to inhibit vestibular-induced eye movements using vision).[28] Vestibular symptom exacerbation indicates a positive test. Positive VOMS testing should prompt referrals for targeted vestibular and vision assessments and rehabilitation.

The King-Devick test is a proprietary, timed saccadic eye movement test requiring individuals to rapidly name numbers, which requires baseline testing.[29-31]

Head Imaging

Mild TBIs are not typically associated with imaging findings that need intervention.[32-36] Severely injured patients with a GCS of 3 to 8 or those who require endotracheal intubation should undergo CT head imaging if they are stable enough to undergo the CT scan. Controversy exists regarding when CT scans are warranted in less-severe head injuries. There are validated criteria to help clinicians determine when to obtain non-contrast head CT, the most common of which are the Canadian CT Head Rule and the New Orleans Criteria. Brain MRI is not commonly indicated in evaluating concussion, however, may have value in cases with atypical or prolonged recovery.[3]

Canadian CT head rule

The "Canadian CT head rule" suggests that there is medium risk of finding radiographic changes in CT if there are following:

1. Amnesia >30 min before impact (retrograde amnesia)
2. A dangerous mechanism (pedestrian struck by motor vehicle, occupant ejected from motor vehicle, and fall from a height of >3 ft or five stairs)

The New Orleans Criteria

The New Orleans Criteria is used to predict which concussed patients are likely to have an intracranial hemorrhage when a head CT has been taken. These criteria recommend that a CT be taken if the following criteria are present:

1. A LOC
2. A GCS of 15
3. Normal findings after a brief neurological examination

And any one of the following:

4. Headache
5. Vomiting
6. Age >60 years
7. Drug or alcohol intoxication
8. Persistent anterograde amnesia (deficits in short-term memory)
9. Evidence of traumatic soft tissue or bone injury above clavicles or seizure (suspected or witnessed)

Blood and Salivary Biomarkers

Biomarkers have the potential in aiding in diagnosis and prognosis of TBI of different severities, including concussion. Blood biomarkers may denote processes such as neuronal injury, glial injury, axonal injury, and inflammation (**Table 1**).[37] Glial and neuronal biomarkers glial fibrillary acidic protein (GFAP) and serum ubiquitin C-terminal hydrolase-L1 (UCH-L1) are associated with severity of concussion and intracranial lesions in children and youth[38,39].

Salivary microRNA (miRNA) and salivary extracellular vesicles can serve as minimally invasive tools to assess TBI symptoms, and may increase the accuracy of diagnosis in mild TBI.[40] Studies have also shown a lower salivary melatonin production in the months to years post-TBI.[41,42]

MANAGEMENT OF CONCUSSION

Current consensus guidelines recommend 24 to 48 hours of symptom-limited cognitive and physical rest, followed by a gradual increase in activity, staying below symptom-exacerbation thresholds.[3]

Physical Activity

There is growing evidence that early sub-symptom threshold aerobic exercise speeds up recovery in sports-related concussions and reduces the risk for persistent post-concussive symptoms.[43–46] The beneficial effects of exercise may be explained by improved autonomic nervous system balance and carbon dioxide sensitivity, increased CBF, upregulation of brain-derived neurotrophic factor gene, and positive effects on mood and sleep.[47–51] Providers should consider prescribing mild-to-moderate aerobic exercise following sports-related concussion.

Cognitive Activity and Screen Time

Cognitive work should be modified or limited to that which does not exacerbate symptoms.[52] Limiting and avoiding screen time during the first 48 hours of concussion recovery may shorten duration of concussive symptoms. More research is needed to quantify safe doses and types of screen time, and to determine whether avoiding screen time beyond 48 hours would have additional benefits.[53]

Targeting Symptoms

The majority of concussion symptoms will resolve spontaneously. The mainstay of concussion management is identifying symptom triggers and targeting specific symptoms. Management options include cervical physical therapy, vestibular and oculomotor therapy, cognitive rehabilitation, cognitive-based therapy, and medications.[44] It is important to understand how symptoms of concussion interact and consider holistic and multidisciplinary approaches to treatment (**Table 2**).

Table 1
Blood and salivary biomarkers

Event	TBI Biomarker	Clinical Utility
Neuronal cell injury	Serum neuron-specific enolase (NSE), a neuronal cytoplasmic enzyme Serum ubiquitin C-terminal hydrolase-L1 (UCH-L1), a neuronal cytoplasmic protein	NSE rises within the first 12 h after TI and declines within hours or days. Hemolysis also increases serum NSE limiting its specificity. UCH-L1 rises within the first 6–24 h following TBI, likely due to break down of the blood–brain barrier and has been found to correlate with TBI severity.
Glial cell injury	S100B, a glial cell protein GFAP, an intermediate filament in astroglial cells	S100B can be used as a prognostic biomarker after TBI and has been correlated with post-concussive symptoms. However, S100B can also be released by skeletal muscles, cardiac muscle, and adipose tissue, and may not be accurate at predicting long-term outcomes. GFAP increases following TBI and may be used to stratify risk for developing cognitive and psychiatric disabilities.
Axonal injury	Neurofilament proteins (NFs), neuronal and axonal proteins Myelin basic protein (MBP), a marker of axonal injury Tau, a microtubule-associated protein expressed on neurons, which forms neurofibrillary tangles when hyperphosphorylated	NF release may predict chronic morbidity and cognitive disability following TBI. MBP release is delayed and non-specific for CNS injury, limiting its utility for accurate diagnosis and prognosis Tau hyperphosphorylation occurs in the setting of TBI-related cerebral ischemia. Studies show mixed utility of serum tau in predicting TBI severity and clinical outcome. CSF tau is more accurate.
Extracellular vesicles	Extracellular vesicles (EVs), membranous particles secreted by cells to aid in intercellular communication	EVs, including exosomes and microRNA (miRNA), are promising biomarkers for TBI, and may be more feasible to isolate.
Inflammation	Inflammatory cytokines, IL-1, IL-6, IL-8, IL-10, and TNF-α, are released from activated microglia and leukocytes following TBI	Prolonged release of cytokines contributes to neurodegenerative disease, and elevated levels may correlate with injury severity, however, are non-specific.

Table 2
Therapy options targeting specific concussion symptoms

Therapy	When to Consider	Therapy Details
Cervical physical therapy	Cervical symptoms and exam findings Tension-type headaches	Physical therapy treatments typically involve manual therapy techniques, proprioceptive (head position sense) retraining, stabilization exercises, and anti-inflammatory modalities
Vestibular and oculomotor therapy	Vestibular and ocular symptoms and exam findings	Balance retraining Oculomotor retraining
Cognitive-based therapy	Depression or anxiety interfering with work or school Athletes struggling with time out of playing sport	
Sleep restoration	Irregular sleep schedule Difficulty falling asleep Difficulty staying asleep	Sleep hygiene practices Cognitive behavioral therapy for insomnia (CBT-i)
Symptom-targeted medications	Prolonged symptoms	*Headache* Riboflavin, coenzyme Q-10, and magnesium oxide Acetaminophen or Tylenol (caution to avoid overuse or rebound headaches) Triptans Beta-blockers Calcium channel blockers Topiramate *Mood* SSRI or other mood stabilizers *Sleep* Melatonin Hypnotic medications for short-term use only

(Data from Leddy JJ, Haider MN, Ellis M, Willer BS. Exercise is Medicine for Concussion. Curr Sports Med Rep. 2018;17(8):262-270.)

Returning to Activities

As symptoms from concussion improve, it is helpful to have a framework to return to school and sports (**Boxes 3** and **4**). Student athletes should be encouraged to return to school tasks and classes before returning to sports. A return to sport must follow a stepwise protocol, during which symptoms and concussion signs are assessed routinely. Driving requires cognitive, visual, and motor skills, all of which can be affected by sports-related concussions. Although no widely accepted return-to-driving protocols exist, it is important to discuss the potential risks of driving with athletes and limit driving and other cognitively intensive tasks accordingly.

Athletes with complicated or prolonged recovery may require a multidisciplinary team with specific expertise across the scope of concussion management. Clinicians should individualize adjustments based on patient-specific symptoms, symptom severity, academic demands, as well as pre-existing conditions, such as mood disorder, learning disability, or attention-deficit/hyperactivity disorder.

MANAGEMENT OF CONVULSING ATHLETE

Most convulsive episodes terminate within 2 to 3 minutes of onset. During this time, the athlete should be closely observed while ensuring to create as safe an environment as possible by loosening tight clothing, helping the individual to the ground and on their side, and removing any hazardous objects. Prolonged convulsive episodes

---

Box 3
Return to learn

Facilitate communication and transition back to school
- Notify school personnel after injury to prepare for return to school.
- Obtain consent for communication between medical and school teams.
- Designate point person to monitor the student's status related to academics, recovery, and coping with injury, and communicate with the medical team.
- School health professional, guidance counselor, administrator, athletic trainer.
- Develop a plan for missed assignments and exams.
- Adjust schedule to accommodate reduced or modified attendance if needed.

Classroom adjustments
- Breaks as needed during school day.
- Reduce class assignments and homework.
- Allow increased time for completion of assignments and testing.
- Delay exams until student is adequately prepared and symptoms do not interfere with testing.
- Allow testing in a separate, distraction-free environment.
- Modify due dates or requirements for major projects.
- Provide preprinted notes or allow peer notetaker.
- Avoid high-risk or strenuous physical activity.

School environment adjustments
- Allow use of headphones/earplugs to reduce noise sensitivity.
- Allow use of sunglasses/hat to reduce light sensitivity.
- Limit use of electronic screens or adjust screen settings, including font size, as needed.
- Allow student to leave class early to avoid crowded hallways.
- Avoid busy, crowded, or noisy environments—music room, hallways, lunch room, vocational classes, assemblies.

(Reproduced from Harmon KG, Clugston JR, Dec K, et al. American Medical Society for Sports Medicine position statement on concussion in sport. Br J Sports Med. 2019;53(4):213-225.)

> **Box 4**
> **Return to sport**
>
> *Stage 1*: Symptom-limited activity
>
> Reintroduction of normal activities of daily living. Symptoms should not worsen with activity.
>
> *Stage 2*: Light aerobic exercise
>
> Walking, stationary biking, controlled activities that increase heart rate.
>
> *Stage 3*: Sport-specific exercise
>
> Running, skating, or other sport-specific aerobic exercise avoiding risk of head impact.
>
> *Stage 4*: Non-contact training drills
>
> Sport-specific, non-contact training drills that involve increased coordination and thinking. Progressive introduction of resistance training.
>
> *Stage 5*: Full contact practice, return to normal training activities. Assess
>
> psychological readiness.
>
> *Stage 6*: Return to sport
>
> Each stage is generally 24 hours without the return of concussion symptoms.

require urgent medical care and transportation to an appropriate medical facility. If the convulsion lasts 5 minutes or longer, administration of a benzodiazepine should be considered if available. The preferred route of administration is rectal, however, buccal spray is also an option. It also is important to rule out hypoglycemia, intracranial bleeding or pathology, and other causes of non-traumatic seizure. Once convulsions have ceased, the athlete should be transferred to the emergency department, where a thorough workup can be done. Prophylaxis with an anticonvulsant, typically levetiracetam, may prevent early PTE, and is generally recommended for penetrating brain injuries.

CLINICS CARE POINTS

- Head injuries represent an important injury designation, for which sports medicine providers should be prepared to recognize, manage, and appropriately triage
- Intracranial hemorrhage represents an important subset of head injury that requires early identification and variable triage, based on clinical and imaging findings.
- Concussions represent a form of mild TBI, with both physiologic and short-term clinical impacts and require careful management before return to play.
- On-field evaluation of head injuries requires a stepwise process for evaluating airway, breathing, circulation, disability, and trauma (ABCDE).
- Standardized evaluation tools for concussion, including the SCAT-5, King-Devick, and VOMS, for concussion are important in assessing readiness for return to play.
- Early submaximal exercise may hasten return to sport, as evidence around concussion management continues to evolve.
- The outcomes of TBI, while historically associated with changes in cognition, movement, and speech, are controversial, and in recent years, mental health concerns have been identified as a potential co-variable for concussion outcomes.

DISCLOSURE

No financial disclosures.

REFERENCES

1. Harmon KG, Drezner JA, Gammons M, et al. American Medical Society for Sports Medicine position statement: concussion in sport. Br J Sports Med 2013;47(1):15–26, published correction appears in Br J Sports Med. 2013 Feb;47(3):184.
2. CDC. Traumatic Brain Injury & Concussion. 2022. Available at: https://www.cdc.gov/traumaticbraininjury/concussion/symptoms.html. Accessed March 28, 2023.
3. Harmon KG, Clugston JR, Dec K, et al. American Medical Society for Sports Medicine position statement on concussion in sport. Br J Sports Med 2019;53(4): 213–25.
4. Hyden A, Tennison M. Evaluation and management of sports-related lacerations of the head and neck. Curr Sports Med Rep 2020;19(1):24–8.
5. Almulhim AM, Madadin M. Scalp laceration. Treasure Island (FL): StatPearls Publishing; 2022. StatPearls.
6. Rajashekar D, Liang JW. Intracerebral hemorrhage. Treasure Island (FL): StatPearls Publishing; 2022. StatPearls.
7. Panourias IG, Skiadas PK, Sakas DE, et al. Hippocrates: a pioneer in the treatment of head injuries. Neurosurgery 2005;57(1):181–9.
8. Mesfin FB, Gupta N, Hays Shapshak A, et al. Diffuse axonal injury. Treasure Island (FL): StatPearls Publishing; 2022. StatPearls.
9. Hinson HE, Rowell S, Schreiber M. Clinical evidence of inflammation driving secondary brain injury: a systematic review. J Trauma Acute Care Surg 2015;78(1): 184–91.
10. Mrozek S, Vardon F, Geeraerts T. Brain temperature: physiology and pathophysiology after brain injury. Anesthesiol Res Pract 2012;2012:989487.
11. Schneider RC. Football head and neck injury. Surg Neurol 1987;27(5):507–8.
12. Wetjen NM, Pichelmann MA, Atkinson JLD. Second Impact Syndrome: Concussion and Second Injury Brain Complications, 211. American College of Surgeons; 2010. p. 553–7.
13. McLendon LA, Kralik SF, Grayson PA, et al. The controversial second impact syndrome: a review of the literature. Pediatr Neurol 2016;62:9–17.
14. Engelhardt J, Brauge D, Loiseau H. Second impact syndrome. Myth or reality? Neurochirurgie 2021;67(3):265–75.
15. Najafi MR, Tabesh H, Hosseini H, et al. Early and late posttraumatic seizures following traumatic brain injury: a five-year follow-up survival study. Adv Biomed Res 2015;4:82.
16. Annegers JF, Hauser WA, Coan SP, et al. A population-based study of seizures after traumatic brain injuries. N Engl J Med 1998;338(1):20–4.
17. Smith DH, Johnson VE, Trojanowski JQ, et al. Chronic traumatic encephalopathy - confusion and controversies. Nat Rev Neurol 2019;15(3):179–83.
18. Marshall LF, Gautille T, Klauber MR, et al. The outcome of severe closed head injury. J Neurosurg 1991;75(Supplement):S28–36.
19. Chesnut RM, Marshall LF, Klauber MR, et al. The role of secondary brain injury in determining outcome from severe head injury. J Trauma 1993;34(2):216–22.
20. Healey C, Osler TM, Rogers FB, et al. Improving the Glasgow Coma Scale score: motor score alone is a better predictor. J Trauma 2003;54(4):671–80.

21. Mills BM, Conrick KM, Anderson S, et al. Consensus recommendations on the prehospital care of the injured athlete with a suspected catastrophic cervical spine injury. J Athl Train 2020;55(6):563–72.
22. Gale SD, Decoster LC, Swartz EE. The combined tool approach for face mask removal during on-field conditions. J Athl Train 2008;43(1):14–20.
23. Lam BL, Thompson HS, Corbett JJ. The prevalence of simple anisocoria. Am J Ophthalmol 1987;104(1):69–73.
24. Magee DJ, Manske RC. Chapter 18: emergency sports assessment. In: Orthopedic physical assessment. 7th ed. St. Louis, MO: Elsevier; 2021. p. 1215–40.
25. Chin EY, Nelson LD, Barr WB, et al. Reliability and validity of the sport concussion assessment tool-3 (SCAT3) in high school and collegiate athletes. Am J Sports Med 2016;44(9):2276–85.
26. Garcia GP, Broglio SP, Lavieri MS, et al. CARE consortium investigators. Quantifying the value of multidimensional assessment models for acute concussion: an analysis of data from the NCAA-DoD care consortium. Sports Med 2018;48(7): 1739–49.
27. Valovich McLeod TC, Hale TD. Vestibular and balance issues following sport-related concussion. Brain Inj 2015;29(2):175–84.
28. Mucha A, Collins MW, Elbin RJ, et al. A brief vestibular/ocular motor screening (VOMS) assessment to evaluate concussions: preliminary findings. Am J Sports Med 2014;42(10):2479–86.
29. Leong DF, Balcer LJ, Galetta SL, et al. The King-Devick test for sideline concussion screening in collegiate football. J Optom 2015;8(2):131–9.
30. Valle Alonso J, Fonseca Del Pozo FJ, Vaquero Álvarez M, et al. Comparison of the Canadian CT head rule and the New Orleans criteria in patients with minor head injury in a Spanish hospital. Med Clin 2016;147(12):523–30.
31. Mori K, Abe T, Matsumoto J, et al. Indications for computed tomography in older adult patients with minor head injury in the emergency department. Acad Emerg Med 2021;28(4):435–43.
32. Ibañez J, Arikan F, Pedraza S, et al. Reliability of clinical guidelines in the detection of patients at risk following mild head injury: results of a prospective study. J Neurosurg 2004;100(5):825–34.
33. Smits M, Dippel DW, de Haan GG, et al. External validation of the Canadian CT head rule and the new orleans criteria for CT scanning in patients with minor head injury. JAMA 2005;294(12):1519–25.
34. Ghaith HS, Nawar AA, Gabra MD, et al. A literature review of traumatic brain injury biomarkers. Mol Neurobiol 2022;59(7):4141–58.
35. Stiell 2005
36. Haydel 2000
37. Ghaith 2021
38. Papa L, Rosenthal K, Cook L, et al. Concussion severity and functional outcome using biomarkers in children and youth involved in organized sports, recreational activities and non-sports related incidents. Brain Inj 2022;36(8):939–47.
39. Papa L, Ladde JG, O'Brien JF, et al. Evaluation of glial and neuronal blood biomarkers compared with clinical decision rules in assessing the need for computed tomography in patients with mild traumatic brain injury. JAMA Netw Open 2022;5(3):e221302.
40. Porteny J, Rovar E, Lin S, et al. Salivary biomarkers as indicators of TBI diagnosis and prognosis: a systemcatic review. Mol Diagn Ther 2022;26:169–87.
41. Shekleton JA, Parcel DL, Redman JR, et al. Sleep disturbance and melatonin levels following traumatic brain injury. Neurology 2010;74:1732–8.

42. Grima NA, Ponsford JL, St Hilaire MA, et al. Circadian melatonin rhythm following traumatic brain injury. Neurorehabil Neural Repair 2016;30:972–7.
43. Leddy JJ, Haider MN, Ellis M, et al. Exercise is medicine for concussion. Curr Sports Med Rep 2018;17(8):262–70.
44. Leddy JJ, Master CL, Mannix R, et al. Early targeted heart rate aerobic exercise versus placebo stretching for sport-related concussion in adolescents: a randomised controlled trial. Lancet Child Adolesc Health 2021;5(11):792–9.
45. Cordingley DM, Cornish SM. Efficacy of aerobic exercise following concussion: a narrative review. Appl Physiol Nutr Metab 2023;48(1):5–16.
46. Cordingly 2022
47. Besnier F, Labrunée M, Pathak A, et al. Exercise training-induced modification in autonomic nervous system: an update for cardiac patients. Ann Phys Rehabil Med 2017;60(1):27–35.
48. Erickson KI, Voss MW, Prakash RS, et al. Exercise training increases size of hippocampus and improves memory. Proc Natl Acad Sci U S A 2011;108(7):3017–22.
49. Nass RD, Elger CE, Fink GR, et al. Kommotionelle Konvulsionen: Epileptischer Anfall oder nicht? [Concussive convulsions: seizure or no seizure?]. Fortschr Neurol Psychiatr 2011;79(11):655–9.
50. Kuhl NO, Yengo-Kahn AM, Burnette H, et al. Sport-related concussive convulsions: a systematic review. Phys Sportsmed 2018;46(1):1–7.
51. Szaflarski JP, Nazzal Y, Dreer LE. Post-traumatic epilepsy: current and emerging treatment options. Neuropsychiatr Dis Treat 2014;10:1469–77.
52. Schneider KJ, Iverson GL, Emery CA, et al. The effects of rest and treatment following sport-related concussion: a systematic review of the literature. Br J Sports Med 2013;47(5):304–7.
53. Macnow T, Curran T, Tolliday C, et al. Effect of screen time on recovery from concussion: a randomized clinical trial. JAMA Pediatr 2021;175(11):1124–31.

Acute and Emergent Spinal Injury Assessment and Treatment

Ron Courson, ATC, PT, SCS, NRAEMT, CSCS[a,*], Barry P. Boden, MD[b],
Jim Ellis, MD[c,d], Glenn Henry, MA, PMDC[a],
Robb Rehberg, PhD, ATC, NREMT[d,e]

KEYWORDS

- Cervical spine injury • Spinal cord injury • Spinal motion restriction
- Emergency action plan

KEY POINTS

- Health care professionals should review and rehearse a variety of transfer techniques. Effective communications should be delivered with clear and concise commands during the motion restriction and transfer techniques.
- Commands for transfer techniques should be given by the rescuer stabilizing the head and cervical spine. This avoids any confusion on who is in charge and all rescuers will focus on this individual for direction.
- The log roll technique is used for prone athletes and is an option for supine athletes. The multi-person lift and the scoop stretcher may be used to lift the supine athlete from the field. Recent research of the multi-person lift has demonstrated that this technique is associated with less cervical motion in cadavers with unstable spines.
- The number of people and transfer technique selected to move a spine-injured athlete should be determined by the medical professional in charge at the scene and the resources available.
- Equipment may be removed either in the hospital emergency department or on-site. Equipment removal on-site allows for application of cervical collar and facilitates physician evaluation in the hospital emergency department and diagnostic testing on arrival. Safe equipment removal requires trained and experienced rescuers.

[a] Sports Medicine, University of Georgia, 1 Selig Circle, Butts-Mehre Hall, Athens, GA 30603, USA; [b] The Orthopaedic Center, a Division of Centers for Advanced Orthopaedics, 14995 Shady Grove Road, Suite 350, Rockville, MD 20815, USA; [c] United States Football League, Birmingham, AL, USA; [d] National Football League, 345 Park Avenue, New York, NY 10154, USA; [e] William Paterson University, 300 Pompton Road, Wayne, NJ 07470, USA
* Correspoding author.
E-mail address: rcourson@sports.uga.edu

Clin Sports Med 42 (2023) 491–514
https://doi.org/10.1016/j.csm.2023.02.011
0278-5919/23/© 2023 Elsevier Inc. All rights reserved.

INTRODUCTION

Sports participation is a leading cause of catastrophic cervical spine injury (CSI) in the United States. Appropriate prehospital care for athletes with suspected CSIs should be available at all levels of sport.[1] The purpose of this article is to review the new consensus statements developed by the Spine Injury in Sport Group: "Consensus Recommendations on the Prehospital Care of the Injured Athlete with a Suspected Catastrophic Cervical Spine Injury"[1] as well as "Best Practices and Current Care Concepts in Prehospital Care of the Spine-Injured Athlete in American Tackle Football."[2] These two manuscripts may be found at https://www.nata.org/practice-patient-care/health-issues/spine-injury along with a video produced by the Sports Institute at University of Washington (UW) Medicine, "Spine Injuries in Sports–Managing On-Field Cervical Spine Injuries."

EPIDEMIOLOGY

Although most spine injuries in sports are minor, a small percentage can result in catastrophic injury with permanent disability or fatality. In the United States, approximately 7% to 9% of all new cases of spinal cord injury (SCI) are secondary to athletic activities.[3,4] Permanent SCI is much more likely to result from cervical spinal injury than thoracic or lumbar injury. Unstable fractures and dislocations are the most common cause of catastrophic cervical spine trauma in athletes and usually occur in the lower cervical spine, especially at C5–C6.[5,6] The spinal cord occupies less than half of the spinal canal's cross-sectional area at the level of the atlas, but close to 75% at the lower cervical levels.[7] Injuries to the mid-level cervical spinal cord region (C3–C5) can damage the motor neuron activation of the phrenic nerve, thus impairing diaphragm muscle contractions and compromising respiration.[8] Catastrophic cervical SCI rarely results in acute sudden death, but the risk of death increases when the injury involves the upper cervical spine.

Sports with the highest risk of SCI in the United States are football, rugby, ice hockey, diving, baseball, cheerleading, equestrian, gymnastics, pole vault, skiing, snowboarding, swimming, and wrestling.[7,9–13] American football has the highest number of catastrophic spine injuries for all sports.[6,9] Although the number of injuries is higher in high school football, the incidence is higher in college football participants likely due to larger players colliding with greater forces.[6] Worldwide the sport resulting in the greatest number of SCIs in the most countries is diving with rugby claiming the highest proportion of SCI caused by any one sport.[12] According to the US National Spinal Cord Injury Statistical Center, the most frequent neurological outcome at hospital discharge for individuals with a sport-related SCI from 1973 to 2013 was incomplete quadriplegia (46.9%), followed by complete quadriplegia (37.4%), incomplete paraplegia (5.9%), and complete paraplegia (5.7%).[3]

The most common mechanism responsible for cervical SCI in sports is an axial force to the crown of the head with the neck slightly flexed. The identification of this mechanism and the ensuing rule changes has dramatically reduced the incidence of injury. In football, early research by Torg and colleagues[5] demonstrated spear tackling, intentional striking of an opponent with the crown of the helmet, as the primary cause for quadriplegia in football and led to the rule banning the tackling technique in the mid-1970s. This ban significantly reduced quadriplegia injuries in college and high school (HS) football. Specifically, in 1976, there were 34 reports of quadriplegia at the HS and college levels and, after the rule change this number decreased to an average of 6 to 10 incidents per year. Owing to the persistent[6] rate of quadriplegia the rules committees strengthened the spear tackling rule, effective in the 2005 to

2006 academic year by removing the word "intentional." The goal of the rule change was to make it easier for referees to call the spear tackling penalty.[6] This rule change as well as the new rules to decrease the number of kickoff returns has the potential to further reduce the number of catastrophic cervical injuries in football.

Similar rule changes focused on reducing axial compression injuries and cervical SCI have been adopted in other sports. In ice hockey, most catastrophic cervical injuries are caused by checking from behind forcing the players head to contact the boards in the vulnerable position. Rules against pushing or checking from behind have reduced the occurrence of these injuries in ice hockey.[14,15] In rugby, catastrophic cervical injuries usually occur during the scrum to the hooker or central player.[16] New rules promoting a sequential or uncontested engagement in rugby have been effective at reducing the incidence of catastrophic cervical spine injuries.[17] In diving, most cervical SCI occur when an athlete dives head first into the shallow end of the pool.[7,18] During regulated diving competitions, a minimum depth at the starting end of the pool can reduce injuries.[7] For recreational diving injuries, interventions include avoiding alcohol intake before swimming/diving, marking swimming depths, and clearly marking spaces that are unsafe to swim or dive.[18]

EMERGENCY ACTION PLAN

Emergency preparation before the event is essential to optimize proper care when dealing with a potential life-threatening situation such as a spine injury. Athletic programs should have an emergency action plan (EAP) developed in conjunction with the local emergency medical services (EMS) agency. Spine injuries are unpredictable and can occur any time during practice or competition. A proper management of emergencies in athletics is critical. The development of the EAP should be a collaborative effort including the sports medicine team, local EMS personnel, and others involved in helping provide emergency care to the injured athlete.[19,20] A separate protocol for the spine-injured athlete should be developed for each sport venue.

The EAP should be approved by the medical director before the beginning of the season. In addition, the EAP should be reviewed and rehearsed by all stakeholders at least annually. This allows all team members, including EMS representation, to be educated on the specific spine management procedures including scenario-based training (eg, athlete in prone or supine position, barriers/space restrictions, the combative athlete, emesis, respiratory and/or cardiac arrest, limited rescuers on-site), maintaining emergency equipment and supplies, selecting personnel, and creating, practicing, and implementing an EAP.[2,19,20] It is recommended that the sports medicine team review each emergency response post-incident for quality improvement purposes.[2]

MEDICAL TIME OUT

Sports medicine teams should conduct a pre-event "Medical Time Out" before each athletic event with medical personnel from both teams, EMS personnel, and the game officials. In order to prevent potentially catastrophic error due to miscommunication, information sharing as well as team and skill coordination among the emergency medical providers is critical components of emergency medical care and the obligation of the host institution/organization. The "Medical Time Out" (**Figs. 1** and **2**) should include a review of items such as medically qualified personnel on-site, equipment available, management protocols for suspected catastrophic injuries, medical professional in charge of the response, signals and communication, contact numbers to local facilities, EMS response routes (primary and secondary), transport procedures, and local hospital trauma management plans. The host medical staff should communicate

- **Introduction**
- **Emergency Personnel Review**
  - Physicians
  - Athletic Trainers
  - EMS
  - X-ray technicians
- **Communication**
  - Emergency Signal: clenched fist held overhead
  - Radios: host medical staff, EMS, x-ray
- **Review Venue Emergency Action Plan**
  - Emergency equipment locations
  - EMS location: emergency cart and ambulance
- **Emergency Review**
  - cardiac, airway, c-spine, exertional heat illness
- **Transport Medical Facility:**
  - Piedmont Athens Regional Med. Ctr. (Level II Trauma Ctr)
  - 1199 Prince Avenue Athens, GA 30606
  - Switchboard: 706- 475-7000
  - ED 706-475-3304
- **SEC Medical Observer Program**
  - Andy Massey xxx-xxx-xxxx
  - Pagers and sideline phone

- **Emergency Contacts:**

Athletic Training Staff: Mobile #

Ron Courson	xxx-xxx-xxxx	Dir. of Sports Med
Drew Willson	xxx-xxx-xxxx	Assoc.Athletic Trainer
Chris Blaszka	xxx-xxx-xxxx	Asst. Athletic Trainer
Brittany deCamp	xxx-xxx-xxxx	Asst. Athletic Trainer
Ryan Madaleno	xxx-xxx-xxxx	Asst. Athletic Trainer
Connor Norman	xxx-xxx-xxxx	Dir. of Rehabilitation

Medical Staff:

Fred Reifsteck, MD	xxx-xxx-xxxx	Primary care/SM
Robert Hancock, MD	xxx-xxx-xxxx	Orthopedic
Eric Gordon, MD	xxx-xxx-xxxx	Orthopedic
Stephen White, MD	xxx-xxx-xxxx	Orthopedic
Kim Walpert, MD	xxx-xxx-xxxx	Neurosurgeon
David Sailors, MD	xxx-xxx-xxxx	Vascular/Internal Med
Stuart Thomas, OD	xxx-xxx-xxxx	Optometrist
David Allen, DMD	xxx-xxx-xxxx	Dentist
Glenn Henry, EMT-P	xxx-xxx-xxxx	Paramedic

Host Sideline Medical Staff:

Mike Dew	xxx-xxx-xxxx	Athletic Trainer
Steve Bryant	xxx-xxx-xxxx	Athletic Trainer

Fig. 1. University of Georgia sports medicine medical timeout checklist.

with visiting team medical personnel for a coordinated emergency approach. This information is important to prepare in advance of events hosted at neutral sites where neither team may be familiar with the venue or local medical facilities.[21,22]

EMERGENCY ASSESSMENT

The initial emergent assessment of the injured athlete on the field of play (FOP) is a critical component in evaluating the player with a suspected cervical spine injury and will guide most of the key medical decisions. All medical evaluations should start with a

Sanford Stadium Address: Gate 6: Players Gate- 260 East Campus Road   Gate 10- 725 S. Lumpkin Street

Venue Directions: Sanford Stadium is located centrally on campus between East Campus Road and Sanford Drive. Two gates provide access to the field of play:
- **Gate 6 Players Gate:** off East Campus Road: follow ramp down to field level (SE corner of stadium)
- **Gate 10:** enter through Tate Student Center parking lot off Lumpkin (cross street Baxter) and follow under Sanford Drive bridge to field level (SW corner of stadium: adjacent to field level First Aid Room)

Roles of First Responders
1. Immediate care of the injured or ill student-athlete(s)
2. Emergency equipment retrieval
3. Communicate with emergency medical system (EMS) on scene
4. Scene control: limit scene to first aid providers and move bystanders away

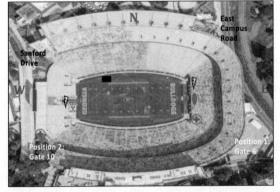
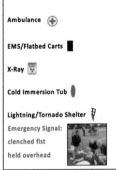

Fig. 2. University of Georgia sports medicine emergency action plan (football game day).

comprehensive history and physical examination. For a suspected SCI in an athlete on the FOP, the history and physical examination may be truncated, focusing on certain critical components. This can also be complicated if the athlete is unconscious or has any decrease in the level of consciousness given the incidence of cervical spine injuries and concomitant mild traumatic brain injury. The rescuer(s) performing the primary examination should assess the level of consciousness of the athlete using the AVPU nomenclature to determine if the athlete is (1) Alert, (2) responds to Verbal stimuli, (3) responds to Painful stimuli, or (4) Unresponsive.

If the athlete is fully alert and can coherently answer questions, the initial questions should focus on the signs related to cervical spine injury from their perspective—neck pain, numbness, paresthesia, weakness, difficulty breathing, and any transient symptoms that may be decreasing. Specifically, asking the player about the mechanism of injury can help to gauge their recall of the injury and level of consciousness. A significant decreased level of consciousness renders the physical examination of the cervical spine inadequate, and the provider must assume the possibility of SCI and place the player in spinal motion restriction. In the conscious of athlete, the history is completed using a few basic questions, and any warning signs for SCI should lead to a focused physical examination.[23]

The on-field assessment of suspected SCI should be a brief examination starting with inspection and palpation of the cervical spine, followed by a more detailed sensory and motor examination. Part of the inspection should include an evaluation of their breathing given the concern for an upper or mid-level SCI. Often just talking to the player is a good evaluation of their airway and breathing but to get more information a pulse oximeter should be readily available. The sensory examination should at a minimum include light touch and the ability to feel painful stimuli in specific dermatomal patterns. The motor examination on the FOP should be gross motor strength in the upper and lower extremities. Although testing reflexes is valuable information, this can typically wait until after the player is removed from the FOP and a more detailed neurologic assessment can be undertaken.

If the player is placed in spinal motion restriction (SMR) and before they are transported to the hospital, there should be a reassessment of their status with a follow-up examination including airway, breathing, and circulation in addition to a follow-up neurological examination to see if anything has changed. Before loading onto the ambulance, there should be a complete set of vital signs taken including pulse oximetry. The patient should receive constant monitoring enroute to the hospital. One of the many advantages to on-field equipment removal is that it allows for better and more closely scrutinized monitoring.

SCENE CONTROL

It is best practice that the emergency scene be controlled, calm, and orderly to facilitate the best medical care. It has been said that "calm is contagious."[24] Bystanders may be well-intentioned but may cause distractions and interfere with the delivery of care. Maintaining a buffer zone between the athlete and all nonmedical people allows adequate space for the sports medicine team to work and position emergency equipment, carts, and ambulances. Failure to maintain a buffer zone between the injured athlete and nonmedical personnel may not allow adequate space for rescuers to work.

SPINAL MOTION RESTRICTION AND TRANSFER TECHNIQUES

As each patient and each emergency are different, health care professionals should review and rehearse a variety of transfer techniques.[25] As mentioned previously, the method of spinal motion restriction and transfer should be discussed at the Medical Time Out meeting, especially due to the movement toward limiting the use of long spine boards in EMS clinical practice.[26] Effective communications should be delivered with clear and concise commands during the motion restriction and transfer techniques. Commands for transfer techniques should be given by the rescuer stabilizing the head and cervical spine. This avoids any confusion on who is in charge and all rescuers will focus on this individual for direction. The log roll technique is used for prone athletes[27] and is an option for supine athletes (see **Fig. 1**). The scoop stretcher[28] may also be used to lift the supine athlete from the field.[29] Recent research of the multi-person lift[27] has demonstrated that this technique is associated with less cervical motion in cadavers with unstable spines (see **Fig. 2**). The number of people and transfer technique selected to move a spine-injured athlete should be determined by the medical professional in charge at the scene and the resources available. Note that variations exist with transferring techniques (eg, verbal commands, hand positions, board angles, centering techniques).

Multi-Rescuer Lift (Requires a Minimum of Eight Rescuers)

The multi-rescuer lift is used to move a suspected spine-injured athlete from the injury scene to a rigid SMR device (often the long spine board), which can then be lifted onto a stretcher and placed into the transport vehicle.

- Rescuer 1 (positioned at the head) provides manual in-line stabilization of the head and cervical spine. Rescuers 2, 3 and 4 and 5, 6 and 7 to position on each side kneeling at the chest, pelvis, and legs to assist with the lift (**Fig. 3**).
- Rescuer 1 gives the commands to direct the others to lift the athlete approximately 6 inches off the ground in unison.
- Rescuer 8 slides the long spine board into place beneath the athlete from the foot end of the athlete (**Fig. 4**).

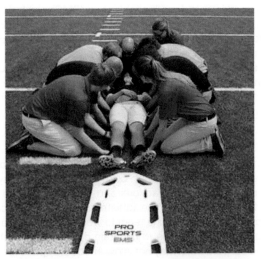

Fig. 3. Multi-person lift technique for supine athlete. (*A*) Rescuer 1 (positioned at the head) provides manual in-line stabilization of the head and cervical spine. Rescuers 2,3 and 4 and 5,6 and 7 position on each side kneeling at the chest, pelvis, and legs) to assist with the lift. (*B*) Rescuer 8 slides the long spine board into place beneath the athlete from the foot end of the athlete.

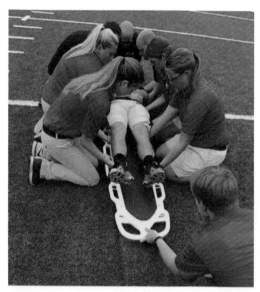

Fig. 4. (B) Rescuer 8 slides the long spine board into place beneath the athlete from the foot end of the athlete.

- Once the SMR device is in position, the athlete is lowered carefully following the commands of Rescuer 1.[30-33]

Supine Log Roll (Requires a Minimum of Five Rescuers)

- Rescuer 1 (positioned at the head) provides manual in-line stabilization of the head and cervical spine (**Fig. 5**).
- Rescuers 2, 3 and 4 assist in rolling athlete.
- On command from Rescuer 1, the athlete is rolled 90° to the side-lying position. Once the patient is in this position Rescuer 5 wedges the long spine board under the athlete at an angle of 45° to the ground.[33-35] On command, the athlete is carefully rolled back to the supine position onto the rigid SMR device.

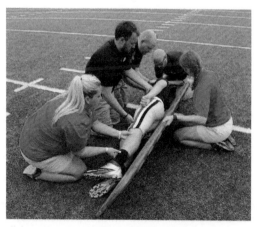

Fig. 5. Supine log roll (requires a minimum of five rescuers).

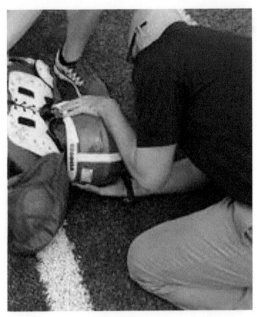

Fig. 6. Rescuer 1 (positioned at the head) provides in-line stabilization of the head and cervical spine using a crossed-hand position.

- If the athlete is not centered on the long spine board, additional adjustments may be needed to shift the patient to the center.
- In some instances, the log roll may be completed with fewer rescuers.[36]

Prone Log Roll Push (Requires a Minimum of Five Rescuers)

- Rescuer 1 (positioned at the head) provides in-line stabilization of the head and cervical spine using a crossed-hand position (**Fig. 6**).
- Rescuers 2, 3 and 4 are positioned along the athlete's body on the same side the athlete's head is facing. The positions of these rescuers are at the athlete's shoulders and chest, the hips, and the legs.

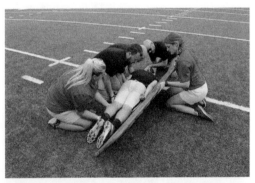

Fig. 7. On command from Rescuer 1, the athlete is slowly rolled away from Rescuers 2, 3 and 4 (ie, pushing) toward the rigid SMR device which is positioned by Rescuer 5 under the athlete at an angle of 45° to the ground.

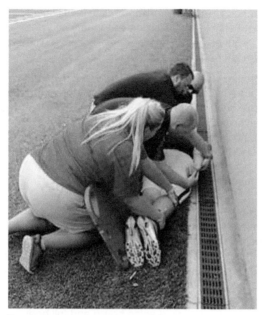

Fig. 8. Prone log roll pull (requires a minimum of four rescuers).

- Rescuer 5 prepares the long spine board.
- On command from Rescuer 1, the athlete is slowly rolled away from Rescuers 2, 3 and 4 (ie, pushing) toward the rigid SMR device, which is positioned by Rescuer 5 under the athlete at an angle of 45° to the ground (**Fig. 7**).
- Once the rigid SMR device is in place, the rescuers readjust their hand position and the athlete is slowly lowered to the rigid SMR device on command of Rescuer 1.[30,31]
- If available, additional rescuers may be used with a hybrid prone log roll pull/push technique with rescuers positioned on both sides.

Prone Log Roll Pull (Requires a Minimum of Four Rescuers)

- (Thumbs toward the face) (**Fig. 8**).
- Rescuers 2, 3 and 4 are positioned along the athlete's body opposite the direction in which the athlete's head is facing. The positions of these rescuers are at the athlete's shoulders and chest, the hips, and the legs.
- On command from Rescuer 1, the athlete is slowly pulled toward Rescuers 2, 3 and 4, whereas the long spine board is positioned against the thighs of the rescuers.
- The athlete is slowly lowered to the rigid SMR device following the commands of Rescuer 1..
- The log roll pull may be used in confined spaces where it is not feasible to position rescuers on both sides of the athlete. If available, additional rescuers may be used.

Centering an Injured Athlete on Spine Board: Once the athlete is transferred onto the spine board, rescuers may need to center the athlete before securing to the spine board. Centering methods that have been used in the past include the horizontal slide, diagonal slide, and the V-adjustment method. A study using cadavers[37] comparing each of the three methods found the horizontal slide best limited cervical spine motion and may be the most helpful for minimizing secondary injury.

Scoop Stretcher (requires a minimum of three rescuers). The scoop stretcher may be used to lift and transfer a supine athlete (**Fig. 9**).

- The scoop stretcher should first be adjusted to the length of the athlete.
- Then, it is separated into two parts at the hinged interlocking device at each end of the scoop stretcher.
- Each of the halves is then wedged under the athlete.
- Rescuer 1 (positioned at the head) stabilizes the head and cervical spine, whereas Rescuers 2 and 3 push the scoop stretcher halves under the athlete until the hinges are latched and in the locked position.[29]
- Care must be taken to not touch the arms of the rescuer 1.

Vacuum immobilization

Vacuum immobilization is used more frequently in Europe than in the United States. The athlete is placed on the vacuum mattress and then the air is removed with a pump while the mattress is molded to the athlete (**Fig. 10A–B**). It has been demonstrated to be more comfortable than the long spine board; however, the long spine board is rigid and cannot suffer failure, such as catastrophic air leak leading to loss of support from the vacuum mattress. If available, vacuum immobilization provides an excellent option for SMR. Full rigid spine board and full body vacuum immobilization are equivalent in the degree of immobilization of the cervical spine.[38,39] Vacuum immobilization may be used with football equipment either on or off.

Packaging

Placing an athlete on an immobilization device in preparation for transportation includes sound packaging techniques. The traditional three-strap technique with chest, pelvis, and thighs allows potential for cephalo-caudal movement on the SMR device. Incorporating an x-strap technique[40] (shoulder/axilla, hips) minimizes cephalo-caudal movement on the immobilization device. This may be accomplished by the use of Velcro spider or X-straps (see **Fig. 10B**) or using speed clip and pin system (**Fig. 11A–C**). The athlete should be centered on the SMR device and body secured, making sure to keep the arms free. The torso is more secure with the strapping system directly to the body. Having the arms free facilitates vital signs and IV access in the ambulance and neurovascular monitoring. The wrists can be secured together if needed with Velcro straps or tape (**Fig. 11D**). The body should always be secured

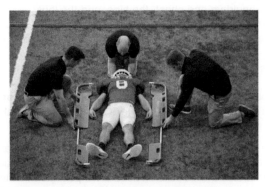

Fig. 9. Scoop Stretcher (requires a minimum of three rescuers).

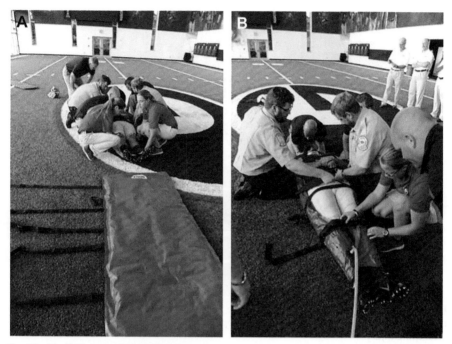

Fig. 10. (*A, B*) Vacuum immobilization.

to the SMR device first and then followed by securing the head. This is important in the event the athlete requires log rolling during the packaging process in order to clear the airway (vomitus or bleeding). If the body is secured to the SMR device, the rescuer can stabilize the head and cervical spine manually during the movement.[2]

A variety of head immobilization devices are available (**Fig. 11**E and F). The head should be stabilized with some form of lightweight block or roll. Weighted blocks such as sandbags are now contraindicated as they have the potential to move the

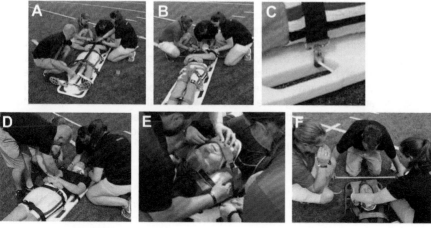

Fig. 11. (*A–F*) Packaging.

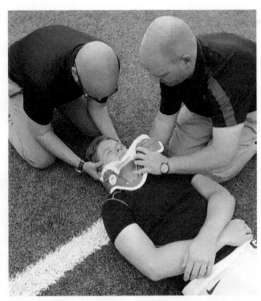

Fig. 12. If the helmet and shoulder pads are removed before transport, a properly fitted rigid cervical stabilization device should be applied to any athlete suspected of having a cervical spine injury.

head laterally if the athlete vomits and must be turned to clear the airway. Tape should be applied to secure the head with two points of contact: (1) eyebrows as landmark for forehead and (2) the chin.[2]

If the helmet and shoulder pads are removed before transport, a properly fitted rigid cervical stabilization device should be applied to any athlete suspected of having a cervical spine injury (**Fig. 12**). With practice, cervical collars can be placed and removed with minimal risk, whereas manual in-line stabilization of the head and neck is maintained.[36] The rigid cervical collar type should be selected in advance. There are many different types of cervical motion restriction devices available on the market. The device should be adjustable or available in various sizes to best fit all athletes. In-line stabilization should be maintained even after application of the device until the athlete is secured properly to an SMR device.[2]

As[41-44] rigid cervical collars are not able to limit cervical spine motion in all planes of movement, manual in-line stabilization should be maintained until the athlete has been stabilized on a full-body SMR device (eg, long spine board, vacuum mattress, and EMS stretcher) and a head stabilization device has been applied. Despite these limitations, cervical collars may reduce cervical motion in patients with potentially unstable spines and still outweigh the disadvantages of their use. The Spinal Motion Restriction in the Trauma Patient—A Joint Position Statement states "An appropriately sized cervical collar is a critical component of SMR and should be used to limit movement of the cervical spine whenever SMR is employed."[45]

EQUIPMENT REMOVAL

Equipment may be removed either in the hospital emergency department or on-site. Equipment removal on-site allows for application of cervical collar and facilitates physician evaluation in the hospital emergency department and diagnostic testing on arrival. Safe equipment removal requires trained and experienced rescuers. If the decision is made to transport the athlete with equipment in place, the facemask should be removed before transportation, regardless of current respiratory status. Tools for facemask removal should be readily accessible, and the availability of a combined tool approach is optimal. If possible, consideration should be given to the use of quick release facemask clips to facilitate facemask removal. Rescuers should be aware that in some instances the facemask cannot be removed, such as some brands of youth football helmets.

Whether the helmet and shoulder pads are removed before transport or at the emergency department, they should be considered a unit and removed. Once the equipment removal process begins, the helmet should be removed first, followed by the shoulder pads. Commands for helmet and shoulder pad removal should be given by the rescuer stabilizing the head and cervical spine.

To remove the helmet, the jersey and then the front of shoulder pads must first be cut, exposing the chest. This allows for one of the rescuers to access and secure c-spine from the front so that the rescuer positioned at the head may remove the helmet. Rescuers should then fit and apply a cervical collar. The athlete should then be secured to a rigid SMR device (ie, EMS stretcher, full body vacuum mattress, scoop stretcher, long spine board, vest type immobilizer).

Helmet Removal Technique (Requires a Minimum of Two Rescuers)

- Rescuer 1 (positioned at the head) stabilizes head and cervical spine.
- Rescuer 2 (positioned at the side of the athlete) cuts helmet chin strap (note that the chin strap should not be unsnapped to avoid any inadvertent head movement). Note that with newer helmet models ear channels, it may not be necessary to remove cheek pads.
- Rescuer 2 cuts jersey and shoulder pads in front with a "T cut": sleeve to sleeve and collar to waist (**Fig. 13**A–B).
- Rescuer 2 assumes cervical spine control from front, allowing Rescuer 1 to release: "I have c-spine control; you can release" (**Fig. 14**A–B).
- Rescuer 2 secures c-spine with an anterior-posterior stabilization technique. The bottom hand carefully cradles the cervical spine and occiput, whereas the top hand grips the chin and jaw, controlling rotation. The top forearm may rest on the athlete's chest providing additional control. This technique allows for a secure hold to stabilize the cervical spine. Previous medial-lateral stabilization techniques where the rescuer grips the side of the athletes' head are limited by the cheek pads inside the helmet(**Fig. 15**A–B). The weight of the head may cause the cervical spine to go into extension when the helmet is removed. The

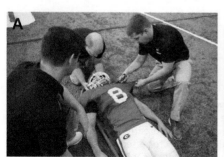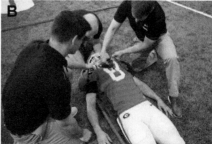

Fig. 13. (*A, B*) Helmet removal technique (requires a minimum of two rescuers).

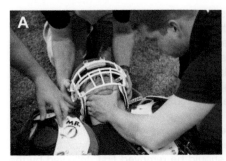
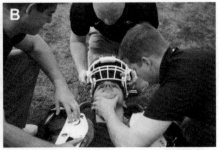

Fig. 14. (*A, B*) Rescuer 2 assumes cervical spine control from front, allowing Rescuer 1 to release: "I have c-spine control; you can release."

anterior-posterior stabilization technique provides additional security to limit cervical extension. Note the medial-lateral stabilization technique may be needed if the posterior hand placement technique causes increase in pain. Putting a posterior hand inside the shoulder pads and on the occiput may put contact points in area of injury especially if there is a deformity. Medial-lateral stabilization technique is still a viable option in some situations. The SM team should practice both anterior-posterior and medial-lateral stabilization and be comfortable with both techniques.

- Rescuer 1 removes helmet; then again assumes cervical spine control, allowing Rescuer 2 to release: "I have c-spine control; you can release."

Shoulder Pad Removal Techniques

Several techniques exist to remove shoulder pads (*following helmet removal*). Rescuers should select the techniques that best fit the individual circumstances associated with each athlete. With the supine athlete, options for shoulder pad removal include:

- Multi-Person Lift (requires a minimum of nine rescuers):
  - Note that helmet has already been removed before shoulder pad removal as described previously

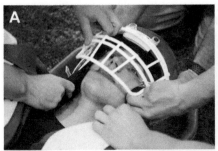
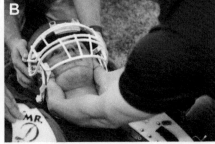

Fig. 15. (*A* and *B*) Rescuer 2 secures c-spine with an anterior-posterior stabilization technique. The bottom hand carefully cradles the cervical spine and occiput, whereas the top hand grips the chin and jaw, controlling rotation. The top forearm may rest on the athlete's chest providing additional control. This technique allows for a secure hold to stabilize the cervical spine. Previous medial-lateral stabilization techniques where the rescuer grips the side of the athletes' head are limited by the cheek pads inside the helmet.

- ○ Rescuer 1 (positioned at the head) stabilizes head and cervical spine
- ○ Before lift, rescuers should cut all shoulder pad straps as well as chest straps and any other straps securing pads to body (eg, rib pads, spider pads, and cervical collars) have been cut, allowing the pads to be removed.
- ○ On command by Rescuer 1, Rescuers 2 - 7 (three on each side) lift athlete approximately 12″ off the ground in unison on command (note that the lift is higher than the standard multi-person lift to allow for shoulder pad clearance during removal).
- ○ Rescuer 8 slides board beneath athlete.
- ○ Rescuer 9 carefully removes shoulder pads without interfering with Rescuer 1's head and cervical spine control.
- ○ Once Rescuer 9 verbalizes "shoulder pads are clear," the athlete is lowered to board on command by Rescuer 1.
- ○ Rescuer 1 maintains cervical spine control, whereas cervical collar is measured and placed on athlete.
- Elevated Torso or "Tilt" Technique (requires a minimum of four rescuers) (**Fig. 16**A–B):
  - ○ Note that helmet has already been removed before shoulder pad removal as described previously.
  - ○ Rescuer 1 (positioned at the head) stabilizes head and cervical spine.
  - ○ Rescuer 2 (positioned at the side of the athlete) assumes cervical spine control from front, allowing Rescuer 1 to release: "I have c-spine control; you can release."
  - ○ Before lift, rescuers should cut all shoulder pad straps as well as chest straps and any other straps securing pads to body (eg, rib pads, spider pads, and cervical collars) have been cut, allowing the pads to be removed.
  - ○ On command by Rescuer 2, Rescuers 3 and 4 carefully lift athlete up, tilting athlete to 30° at waist, similar to the motion of a "sit-up." An alternate method uses one rescuer straddling the athlete to tilt the torso for shoulder pad removal.
  - ○ Rescuer 1 removes shoulder pads from over top of head.

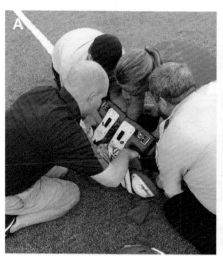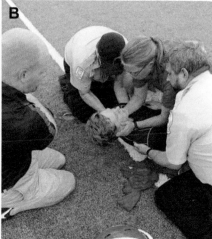

Fig. 16. (*A, B*) Elevated Torso or "Tilt" Technique (requires a minimum of four rescuers).

- o Rescuer 1 then grasps both sides of head and assists Rescuer 2 with cervical spine stabilization as the athlete is lowered down on command by Rescuer 2.
  - o Rescuer 1 then again assumes cervical spine control, allowing Rescuer 2 to release: "I have c-spine control; you can release."
  - o Rescuer 1 maintains cervical spine control, whereas cervical collar is measured and placed on athlete.
  - o Note that the tilt should not be used as a shoulder pad removal technique with suspected concomitant thoracic and/or lumbar injury.[40]
- Flat Torso Technique (requires a minimum of two three rescuers) **Fig. 17**):
  - o Note that helmet has already been removed before shoulder pad removal as described previously).
  - o Rescuer 1 (positioned at the head) stabilizes head and cervical spine.
  - o Rescuer 2 (positioned at the side of the athlete) assumes cervical spine control from front, allowing Rescuer 1 to release: "I have c-spine control; you can release."
  - o The jersey and shoulder pads were previously cut in the front during the helmet removal procedure. Rescuers should cut all shoulder pad straps as well as chest straps and any other straps securing pads to body (eg, rib pads, spider pads, and cervical collars), allowing the pads to be removed.
  - o On command by Rescuer 2, Rescuers 1 and 3 grasp shoulder pads from either side of athlete and carefully slide pads out in an axial direction, whereas Rescuer 2 maintains cervical spine control; this technique may also be executed by one trained rescuer (positioned at the head), carefully sliding pads out while the other rescuer (positioned at the side of the athlete) stabilizes the head and cervical spine.
  - o Rescuer 1 then again assumes cervical spine control, allowing Rescuer 2 to release: "I have c-spine control; you can release."
  - o Rescuer 1 maintains cervical spine control, whereas cervical collar is measured and placed on athlete.

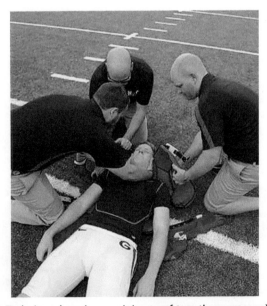

Fig. 17. Flat Torso Technique (requires a minimum of two-three rescuers).

- Log Roll Technique (ideally requires a minimum of five rescuers):
  - Note that helmet has already been removed before shoulder pad removal as described previously)
  - A standard log roll technique is used. Rescuer 1 stabilizes the head and cervical spine.
  - On command by Rescuer 1, Rescuers 2, 3 and 4 perform supine log roll, pausing at the top of the roll.
  - Rescuer 5 cuts the jersey and shoulder pads in back, then positions long spine board and athlete is lowered down onto board on command by Rescuer 1.
  - The jersey and shoulder pads were previously cut in the front during the helmet removal procedure. Rescuers should cut all shoulder pad straps as well as chest straps and any other straps securing pads to body (eg, rib pads, spider pads, and cervical collars), allowing the pads to be removed.
  - The shoulder pads, now separated in both the front and the back, are then removed from each side by Rescuers 2 and 3 on command by Rescuer 1.
  - Rescuer 1 maintains cervical spine control, whereas cervical collar is measured and placed on athlete.
- Quick Release Shoulder Pads (requires a minimum of three rescuers):
  - Some shoulder pads are designed with a quick release mechanism for emergency removal. This involves pulling a cable which separates the shoulder pads in the back.
  - Note that helmet has already been removed before shoulder pad removal as described previously)
  - Rescuer 1 (positioned at the head) stabilizes the head and cervical spine.
  - Rescuer 2 (positioned at the side of the athlete) cuts the emergency quick release tab and pulls a cable releasing the shoulder pads in back.
  - Rescuers should cut all shoulder pad straps as well as chest straps and any other straps securing pads to body (eg, rib pads, spider pads, and cervical collars), allowing the pads to be removed.
  - The shoulder pads, now separated in both the front and the back, are then removed from each side by Rescuers 2 and 3 on command by Rescuer 1
  - Rescuer 1 maintains cervical spine control, whereas cervical collar is measured and placed on athlete.

Over the Head (requires a minimum of four rescuers):

- This technique may be used when it is not possible to cut open the shoulder pads in the front to use any of the above techniques.
- *Note that helmet has already been removed before shoulder pad removal as described previously)*
- Rescuer 1 (positioned at the head) stabilizes the head and cervical spine.
- Before lift, rescuers should cut all shoulder pad straps as well as chest straps and any other straps securing pads to body (eg, rib pads, spider pads, and cervical collars) have been cut, allowing the pads to be removed.
- Rescuer 2 (positioned at the side of the athlete) reaches up under the shoulder pads and take control of the head and cervical spine stabilization from Rescuer 1.
- On command by Rescuer 2, the Elevated Torso or "Tilt" Technique is executed, whereas Rescuer 2 stabilizes the head and cervical spine from the front.
- Rescuers 3 and 4 carefully lift athlete up, tilting athlete to 30° at waist, similar to motion of a "sit-up."
- Rescuer 1 removes shoulder pads from over top of head.
- Rescuer 1 then grasps both sides of head and assists Rescuer 2 with cervical spine stabilization as the athlete is lowered down on command by Rescuer 2.

- Rescuer 1 then again assumes cervical spine control, allowing Rescuer 2 to release: "I have c-spine control; you can release."
- Rescuer 1 maintains cervical spine control, whereas cervical collar is measured and placed on athlete.
- *Note again that the tilt should not be used as a shoulder pad removal technique with suspected concomitant thoracic and/or lumbar injury.*[40]

Regarding options for shoulder pad removal with the prone athlete, the athlete must be log rolled as the multi-rescuer lift-and-slide and scoop stretcher techniques may only be used on supine athletes.[32,37] Rescuers should select either the log roll-push or log roll-pull technique based on the individual circumstances associated with each athlete.

- Rescuer 1 (positioned at the head) stabilizes the head and cervical spine.
- Before initiating the log roll, Rescuer 2 (positioned at the side of the athlete) cuts the jersey and shoulder pads in back and then positions the long spine board.
- On command by Rescuer 1, the log roll procedure is performed by Rescuers 2 - 5 as previously described.
- Once the athlete is rolled to the supine position, the jersey and shoulder pads are cut in the front by Rescuer 2 and the helmet is then removed as previously described.
- Rescuers should cut all shoulder pad straps as well as chest straps and any other straps securing pads to body (eg, rib pads, spider pads, and cervical collars) have been cut, allowing the pads to be removed.
- The shoulder pads, now separated in both the front and the back, are then removed from each side by Rescuers 2 and 3 on command by Rescuer 1.
  ○ Rescuer 1 maintains cervical spine control, whereas cervical collar is measured and placed on athlete.

Other considerations with shoulder pad removal include accessories attached to the shoulder pads such as cervical collars, rib pads, back pads and difficulty or inability to cut pads due to materials involved.

SPECIAL SITUATIONS

Various sports and venues may create special or unique situations that require problem-solving in the event of a spine injury. When managing potential spine injuries in the swimming pool or diving well, the rescuers must coordinate care with lifeguards. Lifeguards have special training with water extraction. Once the athlete is removed safely from the water, the sports medicine team may coordinate care. The gymnastics pit or well also create challenges. The pit is an unstable surface full of foam blocks on the top of a trampoline. The rescuers may position a mat on top of the foam blocks to move closer to the injured gymnast without causing movement (**Fig. 18**). The Kendrick Extrication Device (KED) (**Fig. 19**) may be useful as the gymnast may be in a flexed position. Once the KED is applied, the gymnast may be transferred to a long spine board. The gymnastics well may require additional rescuers to lift the athlete out once packaged.

The pole vault pit in track and field also creates challenges. Again, if the athlete is flexed, application of a KED may facilitate extraction. Closed or confined spaces, such as an athlete positioned against the hockey rink boards or the baseball outfield wall may limit transfer techniques. Rescuers working with these sports should practice scenario-based training with these challenges. Rescuers should also rehearse managing airway distress/arrest, cardiac arrest, and vomiting/airway obstruction.

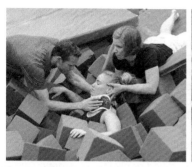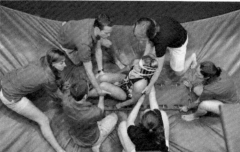

Fig. 18. The Kendrick Extrication Device (KED) can be useful as the gymnast may be in a flexed position.

TRANSPORTATION AND MEDICAL FACILITY CRITERIA

Transportation of the injured or critically ill athlete to the nearest appropriate medical facility is one of the most important decisions in emergency situations in sports. Athletic trainers (ATs), team physicians, and EMS personnel should work collaboratively to ensure that the most appropriate mode of transport and most appropriate destination for potential spinal cord injured patients is chosen. All team medical and athletic training staff should become familiar with local and or state protocols that may predetermine destination. Any deviation from local or state protocols may require on-line medical control intervention.

All potential destinations for transport to medical facilities should be clearly delineated in the EAP and often times may be dependent on the condition of the patient. During the pre-event "Medical Time Out,"[21,22] there must be a specific discussion on transportation destinations for the injured or ill athlete. In sports where cervical spine injury is at greater risk, the primary or secondary hospital designated in the

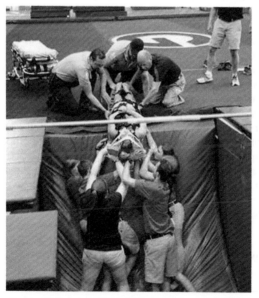

Fig. 19. The gymnastics well may require additional rescuers to lift the athlete out once packaged.

EAP as the "spine" or "neurological" hospital should be specifically named during the "Medical Time Out."

ATs, team physicians, and EMS personnel should determine the most appropriate mode of transport (air vs ground) based on patient condition and distance to the receiving facility. If air medical transport is necessary, predetermined landing zones and global positioning system (GPS) coordinates should be noted on the EAP.

If feasible, an athlete with a spine injury should be transported to a medical facility that can deliver immediate and definitive care. This includes a cervical spine fracture with or without SCI.[46,47]

Immediate and definitive care for the spine-injured athlete includes the following[2]:

- Emergency department staffed with board-certified or eligible emergency medicine physicians
- Personnel trained in equipment removal with a protocol in place to allow team medical personnel to assist with equipment removal
- Computed tomography and MRI scanning available within 30 minutes of patient arrival
- Spine surgeon consultation in house or available within 30 minutes of patient arrival
- 24/7 operating room access
- Critical care physiologic and neurological monitoring
- Rehabilitation services or a preexisting referral system

In an SCI athlete with neurological deficits, time to the operating room and surgical decompression is a critical component in the outcome of the patient's long-term prognosis. In most cases, patients should be transported to a predetermined trauma center in accordance with local or state EMS protocols. If a trauma center is not immediately available, then the patient should be transported to the closest largest community hospital capable of delivering definitive care. If the SCI patient has an unstable airway or is in cardiac arrest, transport to the closest medical facility is warranted.

However, attempts should be made to avoid this additional delay in definitive care as improved outcomes have been reported with expeditious definitive management.[48] The risk of complications increases when a patient remains on the long spine board for an extended period of time after arrival in the emergency department. Increased tissue interface pressures at the occiput, sacrum, and heel have been reported with prolonged immobilization.[49] Transfers within the emergency department should be kept to a minimum to reduce the chance of causing further injury.

When an AT or team physician is involved in the transport of a spine injured athlete, he or she should offer to assist the emergency department (ED) staff with the athlete's care. Establishing the role of the AT or other medical provider who accompanies the athlete to the emergency department before a season starts is a valuable part of the EAP.[2]

Planning the process of transport for home venues before the start of the season and ensuring that a medical time out occurs at home and away games can reduce complications of transport decisions on the FOP and expedite transport of the spine-injured athlete.

CLINICS CARE POINTS

- Athletic programs should have an emergency action plan (EAP) developed in conjunction with the local emergency medical services (EMS) agency.

- A protocol for the spine-injured athlete should be developed.
- Sports medicine teams should conduct a pre-event "Medical Time Out" before each athletic event with medical personnel from both teams, EMS personnel, and the game officials.
- The emergency scene be controlled, calm, and orderly to facilitate the best medical care.
- As each patient and each emergency are different, health care professionals should review and rehearse a variety of transfer techniques.
- The log roll technique is used for prone athletes and is an option for supine athletes. The multi-person lift and the scoop stretcher may also be used to lift the supine athlete from the field. The number of people and transfer technique selected to move a spine-injured athlete should be determined by the medical professional in charge at the scene and the resources available.
- Placing an athlete on an immobilization device in preparation for transportation includes sound packaging techniques. Incorporating an x-strap technique (shoulder/axilla, hips) minimizes cephalo-caudal movement on the immobilization device. The torso is more secure with the strapping system directly to the body. Having the arms free facilitates vital signs and IV access in the ambulance and neurovascular monitoring. The body should always be secured to the SMR device first and then followed by securing the head.
- If the helmet and shoulder pads are removed before transport, a properly fitted rigid cervical stabilization device should be applied to any athlete suspected of having a cervical spine injury.
- Equipment may be removed either in the hospital emergency department or on-site. Equipment removal on-site allows for application of cervical collar and facilitates physician evaluation in the hospital emergency department and diagnostic testing on arrival. Safe equipment removal requires trained and experienced rescuers.
- If the decision is made to transport the athlete with equipment in place, the facemask should be removed before transportation, regardless of current respiratory status.
- Transportation of the injured or critically ill athlete to the nearest appropriate medical facility is one of the most important decisions in emergency situations in sports. If feasible, an athlete with a spine injury should be transported to a medical facility that can deliver immediate and definitive care.

DISCLOSURE

The Authors have nothing to disclose.

REFERENCES

1. Mills B.M., Conrick K.M., Anderson S., et al., Consensus Recommendations on the Prehospital Care of the Injured Athlete with a Suspected Catastrophic Cervical Spine Injury, J Ath Train, 55 (6), 2020, 563–572.
2. Courson R, Ellis J, Herring S, et al. Best Practices and Current Care Concepts in Prehospital Care of the Spine Injured Athlete in American Tackle Football. J Ath Train 2020;55(6):545–62.
3. National Spinal Cord Injury Statistical Center Annual statistical report for the spinal cord injury model systems—complete public version. Spinal Cord Injury Model Systems. University of Alabama at Birmingham. Alabama. 2013. Available at: https://www.nscisc.uab.edu/PublicDocuments/reports/pdf/2013%20NSCISC %20Annual%20Statistical%20Report%20Complete%20Public%20Version.pdf. Published 2013. Accessed 10 July, 2022.
4. Boden BP, Prior C. Catastrophic Spine Injuries in Sports. Curr Sports Med Rep 2005;4:45–9.

5. Torg JS, Guille JT, Jaffe S. Current concepts review: Injuries to the cervical spine in American football players. J Bone Joint Surg 2002;84-A:112.

6. Boden BP, Tachetti RL, Cantu RC, et al. Catastrophic cervical spine injuries in high school and college football players. Am J Sports Med 2006;34(8):1223–32.

7. Boden BP. Direct catastrophic injury in sports. J Am Acad Ortho Surg 2005;13: 445–53.

8. Nicaise C, Hala TJ, Frank DM, et al. Phrenic motor neuron degeneration compromises phrenic axonal circuitry and diaphragm activity in a unilateral cervical contusion model of spinal cord injury. Exp Neurol 2012;235(2):539–52.

9. Kucera KL and Cantu RC. NCCSIR Thirty-eighth Annual Report. National center for catastrophic sports injury research: fall 1982 –Spring 2020. Chapel Hill (NC): National Center for Sports Injury Research; 2020. Available at: nccsir.unc.edu. Accessed 16 July, 2022.

10. Boden BP, Tacchetti R, Mueller FO. Catastrophic cheerleading injuries. Am J Sports Med 2003;31:881–8.

11. Boden BP, Boden MG, Peter RG, et al. Catastrophic injuries in pole vaulters: a prospective 9-year follow-up study. Am J Sports Med 2012;40:1488–94.

12. Boden BP. Lin W. Young M. Available at: http://www.ncbi.nlm.nih.gov/pubmed? term=Young M[Author]&cauthor=true&cauthor_uid=12435642.

13. Mueller FO. Catastrophic injuries in wrestlers. Am J Sports Med 2002;30:791–5.

14. Tator CH, Carson JD, Edmonds VE. Spinal injuries in ice hockey. Clin Sports Med 1998;17:183–94.

15. Morrissette C, Park JP, Lehman RA, et al. Cervical Spine Injuries in the Ice Hockey Player: Current Concepts in Epidemiology, Management and Prevention. Global Spine J 2021;11(8):1299–306.

16. Wetzler MJ, Akpata T, Laughlin W, et al. Occurrence of cervical spine injuries during the rugby scrum. Am J Sports Med 1998;26:177–80.

17. Gianotti S, Hume PA, Hopkins WG, et al. Interim evaluation of the effect of a new scrum law on neck and back injuries in rugby union. Br J Sports Med 2008;42(6): 427–30.

18. Chan CWL, Eng JJ, Tator CH, et al. and the Spinal Cord Injury Research Evidence Team. Epidemiology of sport-related spinal cord injuries:A systematic review. J Spinal Cord Med 2016;39(3):255–64.

19. Courson RW. Preventing sudden death on the athletic field: the athletic emergency plan. Curr Sports Med Rep 2007;6(2):93–100.

20. Anderson JC, Courson RW, Kleiner DM, et al. National Athletic Trainers' Association position statement: emergency planning in athletics. J Ath Train 2002;37(1): 99–104.

21. Courson R. National athletic trainers' association official statement on athletic health care provider "time outs" before athletic events. 2012. Available at: http://www.nata.org/sites/default/files/TimeOut.pdf.

22. National Football League. 60-Minute Medical Meeting Overview Video. Available at: https://link.edgepilot.com/s/1678bc39/tK7BH9K1c0evOCvgcZZ4sw?u= https://vimeo.com/728988672/c0adb7510b. Published July 11, 2022. Accessed 26 November, 2022.

23. Courson R, Clanton M, Patel H. Emergency Assessment. Athl Ther Today 2005; 10(2):19–23.

24. Denver R. Calm is contagious: can you keep your cool when your team is decision-making under stress? Leadercast Wed site. Available at: https//now. leadercast.com/programs/calm-is-contagious. Published 2019. Accessed 14 November, 2022.

25. Courson RW, Rehberg RS, Monaco MJ. Care concepts in management of the spine-injured athlete. In: Rehberg RS, Konin JG, editors. Sports emergency care: a team approach. 3rd edition. Thorofare, NJ: Slack Inc; 2018. p. 63–88.

26. Feld F. Removal of the long spine board from clinical practice. A historical perspective. J Athl Train 2018;83(8):752–5.

27. Conrad BP, Marchese DL, Rechtine GR, et al. Motion in the unstable cervical spine when transferring a patient positioned prone to a spine board. J Athl Train 2013;48(6):797–803.

28. Krell JM, McCoy MS, Sparto PJ, et al. Comparison of the Ferno scoop stretcher with the long backboard for spinal immobilization. Prehosp Emerg Care 2006; 10(1):46–51.

29. Del Rossi G, Rechtine GR, Conrad BP, et al. Are scoop stretchers suitable for use on spine-injured patients? Am J Emerg Med 2010;28(7):751–6.

30. Conrad BP, Rossi GD, Horodyski MB, et al. Eliminating log rolling as a spine trauma order. Surg Neurol Int 2012;3(Suppl 3):S188–97.

31. Swartz EE, Boden BP, Courson RW, et al. National Athletic Trainers' Association position statement: acute management of the cervical spine-injured athlete. J Athl Train 2009;44(3):306–31.

32. Del Rossi G, Horodyski M, Conrad BP, et al. Transferring patients with thoracolumbar spinal instability: are there alternatives to the log roll maneuver? Spine (Phila Pa 1976) 2008;33(14):1611–5.

33. Del Rossi G, Horodyski M, Powers ME. A comparison of spine-board transfer techniques and the effect of training on performance. J Athl Train 2003;38(3): 204–8.

34. Del Rossi G, Horodyski M, Heffernan TP, et al. Spine-board transfer techniques and the unstable cervical spine. Spine 2004;29(7):E134–8.

35. Del Rossi G, Horodyski M, Kaminski TW. Management of cervical- spine injuries. Int J Athl Ther Train 2002;7(2):46–51.

36. Campbell J. International trauma life support for emergency care providers. 7th edition. Upper Saddle River, NJ: Prentice-Hall; 2012.

37. DuBose DN, Zdziarski LA, Scott N, et al. Horizontal slide creates less cervical motion when centering an injured patient on a spine board. J Emerg Med 2016; 50(5):728–33.

38. Prasarn ML, Hyldmo PK, Zdziarski LA, et al. Comparison of the vacuum mattress versus the spine board alone for immobilization of the cervical spine injured patient: a biomechanical cadaveric study. Spine (Phila Pa 1976) 2017;42(24): E1398–402.

39. Luscombe MD, Williams JL. Comparison of a long spinal board and vacuum mattress for spinal immobilisation. Emerg Med J 2003;20(5):476–8.

40. Mazolewski P, Manix TH. The effectiveness of strapping techniques in spinal immobilization. Ann Emerg Med 1994;23(6):1290–5.

41. Richter D, Latta LL, Milne EL, et al. The stabilizing effect of different orthoses in the intact and unstable upper cervical spine: a cadaver study. J Trauma 2001; 50(5):848–54.

42. Horodyski M, DiPaola CP, Conrad BP, et al. Cervical collars are insufficient for immobilizing an unstable cervical spine injury. J Emerg Med 2011;41(5):513–9.

43. Miller CP, Bible JE, Jegede KA, et al. The effect of rigid cervical collar height on full, active, and functional range of motion during fifteen activities of daily living. Spine (Phila Pa 1976) 2010;35(26):E1546–52.

44. Bearden BG, Conrad BOP, Horodyski M, et al. Motion in the unstable cervical spine: comparison of manual turning and use of the Jackson table in prone positioning. J Neurosureg Spine 2007;7(2):161–4.
45. Fischer PE, Perina DG, DElbridge TE, et al. Spinal motion restriction in the trauma patient – a joint position statement. Prehosp Emerg Care 2018;22(6):659–61.
46. Study, M. D. (2019). Spine injury in sport Group. In person meeting.
47. Force, I.-A. T. (2015). InterAssociation task force on the pre-hosptial care of the suspected spine injured athlete. In person meeting.
48. Harrington DT CM. Transfer TImes to Long. Ann Surg 2005;961–8.
49. WJC HJ. Pain and tissue interface pressures during spine board immobilization. Annuals of Emergency Medicine 1995;26(1):31–6.

Fractures and Dislocations on the Playing Field
Which Are Emergent and What to Do?

James T. Stannard, MD, PhD[a], James P. Stannard, MD[b],*

KEYWORDS

- Fractures • Dislocations • High-energy injuries • Treatment options • Athletes

KEY POINTS

- Timeout with other medical personal prior to competition. Discuss specifics such as equipment available, nearest hospital and ambulance availability.
- Always start with ABCs of trauma. Quickly identify emergent vs non emergent injuries and triage appropriately.
- Be prepared to reduce fractures/dislocation on the field and stabilize as indicated.

INTRODUCTION

Although it is possible to fracture virtually any bone during athletic activities, the most common fractures are listed in the paragraph above. Common emergent fractures include the cervical spine and tibia, and team physicians must have a plan for handling both injuries. Cervical spine fractures are beyond the scope of this article and the expertise of the senior author (J.P.S.) but it is critical to have a plan for caring for patients with suspected cervical injury. Before the athletic competition, the sports medicine physician must know where the spine board and cervical collar are located. It is also essential to determine if equipment such as a helmet will be left on with the facemask removed or if the whole helmet will be removed. Ideally, there should be a "timeout" before the event with all medical personnel to go over these details.

Fracture Demographics

Upper extremity fractures (52.4%) were more common than lower extremity (45.4%) or axial skeleton (2.2%) related fractures in a study evaluating the epidemiology of sports fractures in athletes in Scotland.[1] The most common upper extremity fractures in athletes were phalangeal (204), distal radius (167), metacarpals (125), and then clavicles (98).[2] Ankle fractures represented the most common lower extremity

[a] Department of Orthopaedic Surgery, University of Missouri, 1100 Virginia Avenue, Columbia, MO 65212, USA; [b] Department of Orthopaedic Surgery, Missouri Orthopaedic Institute, University of Missouri, 1100 Virginia Avenue, Columbia, MO 65212, USA
* Corresponding author.
E-mail address: stannardj@health.missouri.edu

Clin Sports Med 42 (2023) 515–524
https://doi.org/10.1016/j.csm.2023.02.012
0278-5919/23/© 2023 Elsevier Inc. All rights reserved.

fracture (92) followed by metatarsal (44) and tibial shaft (24) fractures.[2] Sports most frequently associated with fractures in this European study included soccer (35.5%), rugby (14.5%), and cycling (10.5%).[2] Sports with the highest incidence of fractures vary by geographic area of the world. It is important for a team physician to be aware of the frequency of fractures in the sport they are covering and to have appropriate supplies and emergency transport available for the initial care of these injuries.

PATIENT EVALUATION OVERVIEW AND TREATMENT OPTIONS

Fractures should be grossly realigned by applying traction and then should be immobilized in a splint. Radiographs should be obtained at the stadium if facilities are available, and the athlete should then be transported to a local hospital emergency department for definitive treatment. The nearest hospital with appropriate facilities should be identified before the start of competition. It is also important to have ambulance transport available at the stadium for collision sports whenever possible.

Fractures

Common fractures include ankle, clavicle, and knee osteochondral (OC) fractures. Ankle[3,4] and clavicle fractures are far more common than cervical or tibial fractures in athletes but are usually much less severe and emergent.[5]

Open fractures

There are many other fractures that can occur during athletic competitions. Any open fracture is emergent due to the risk of infection. Athletes with open fractures should be transported to a hospital as quickly as possible. Attempts at irrigation or cleansing of the wound at the site of the athletic competition should not be done if they will delay transport to the definitive treatment facility. With open injuries, it is important to determine tetanus immunization status and immunize as needed.

Tibia fractures

Tibia fractures, both plateau and shaft, are another fracture that is often emergent and can have devastating consequences. Vascular injuries are a concern with both types, with up to 29% of open tibial shaft fractures having a concomitant vascular injury.[5] The frequency of tibial fractures varies by sport, with one publication noting that 22% of lower extremity fractures in Belgian soccer players involve the tibial shaft.[7] Risk factors in that article included older age, male sex, and recreational players (as compared with professional). Initial management involves splinting the fracture, providing wound care if a wound is present, and transporting to the local hospital. Great care must be taken to evaluate the injured athlete with a tibial plateau or shaft fracture sequentially for vascular injury and the development of compartment syndrome.

Tibial fractures can have devastating consequences for the athlete and are a career-threatening injury. A metanalysis reported on return to sport after tibial shaft fractures.[3] Sixteen studies with 889 patients were included in the analysis. Fractures treated surgically had a return-to-sport rate of 92%, whereas those treated nonoperatively had a 67% return-to-sport rate ($P < .01$). Overall, 75% of those treated surgically returned to the same level of sport compared with only 40% in the nonsurgical group. Return to athletics ranged from 12 to 54 weeks after surgery and from 28 to 182 weeks after conservative care. The difference was significant ($P < .01$) and was a mean of 69.5 weeks longer in nonoperatively managed patients.[3] When one considers that the surgically managed group generally had more severe and more displaced fractures, it is clear that careful consideration should be given to surgical management. Tibia fractures

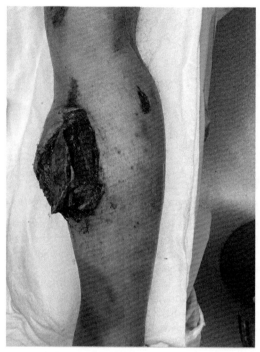

Fig. 1. Open tibia fracture with significant soft tissue injury.

are frequently open and require careful soft tissue management in addition to treating the bone injury (**Fig. 1**).

Osteochondral fractures

OC fractures of the knee are uncommon but represent a unique fracture type because they occur in joints and involve the articular cartilage. Children and adolescents are more susceptible to these injuries because the calcified cartilage layer is incompletely formed.[1] They are most commonly seen in the patella, trochlea, and femoral condyles and should be ruled out following patella dislocations.[1,8] The most common location on the femoral condyle is the lateral aspect of the medial femoral condyle. OC fractures can occur as a contact, or a noncontact injury, and it is important to maintain a high index of suspicion with a knee injury in a pediatric athlete. Initial radiographs may be misleading and miss the injury. In a young athlete with a hemarthrosis and negative radiographs, advanced imaging with MRI should be considered.[1] Although these fractures do not usually represent an emergent injury, they should be treated urgently. Stable and nondisplaced fractures may be treated conservatively.[8] Displaced and unstable fractures normally require surgical treatment with reduction and fixation if possible with large fragments.[1]

Other knee fractures

In addition to OC fractures, there are several fractures around the knee that occur in athletes. These include tibial plateau, supracondylar femur, and patella fractures. The Cleveland Clinic sports clinic reported on a total of 41 fractures around the knee during a 10-year period.[9] Patella fractures represented most of these injuries (73%) followed by tibial plateau (17%), distal femur (5%), and intercondylar eminence

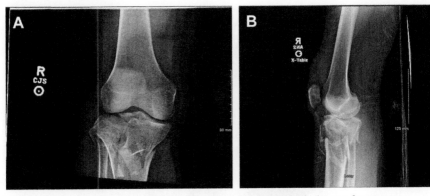

Fig. 2. AP (*A*) and lateral (*B*) radiographs of comminuted tibial plateau fracture.

(5%) fractures. Basketball was the most common sport associated with fractures around the knee (32%), followed by football (20%) and gymnastics (10%). Patella and distal femur fractures rarely represent an emergency injury but tibial plateau fractures must be treated as an emergency until vascular injuries and compartment syndrome are ruled out (**Fig. 2**A, B). Many tibial plateau fractures actually represent a fracture dislocation and are at high risk for these complications.[10] Differentiating between a fracture versus fracture dislocation is very difficult at the athletic venue so it is critical to maintain an extremely high index of suspicion.[8,10] A good vascular and neurologic examination should be documented, as well as an assessment of the lower leg compartments for signs of compartment syndrome. Patients with tibial plateau or distal femur fractures should be immobilized and expeditiously transferred to the hospital for definitive treatment.

Clavicle fractures
Clavicle fractures are relatively common injuries in contact sports.[5] They do not represent an emergency unless the fracture is open, skin is threatened, or has an associated vascular injury. Athletes that sustain a suspected clavicle fracture should be initially treated with a sling or shoulder immobilizer and should be transported to a hospital for definitive care on a nonemergent basis.

Joint Dislocations
Dislocations can occur at large joints such as the shoulder, hip, or knee or can occur at smaller joints of the hand and foot. The severity of these injuries varies significantly and can represent limb-threatening injuries. Recent data in the United States reveals that 2.6 million children (up to age 19) are treated in emergency rooms annually for sports-related injuries. Joint dislocations and separations represent 3.6% of these injuries.[11] The 3 most common joint dislocations were shoulder (54.9%), wrist/hand (16.5%), and knee (16%).[11] These injuries vary in severity but several of them represent orthopedic emergencies. We will discuss evaluation and initial management of these injuries.

Knee dislocations
Dislocations of the tibiofemoral joint represent one of the most serious injuries an athlete can sustain and are an orthopedic emergency (**Fig. 3**). These injuries require an initial assessment of the neurovascular status of the leg, paying particular attention to a good vascular examination. In the hospital setting, either a good distal pulse examination or an ankle brachial index (ABI) is an accepted method of performing an initial assessment of the popliteal artery.[12,13] Examination of the posterior tibial artery

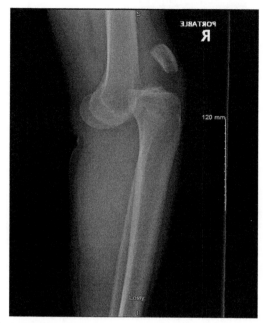

Fig. 3. Radiograph demonstrating right knee dislocation.

and dorsalis pedis pulses have a 75% positive predictive value and a 93% negative predictive value for detecting a significant vascular injury.[14] The key thing for the orthopedic sports provider to remember is that the presence of good pulses does not rule out significant vascular injury due to collateral flow. The absence of pulses nearly always signals limb-threatening popliteal injury. ABI has a better positive predictive value as long it the value is 0.9 or higher.[15] Frequently all of the equipment to perform ABI are not readily available on the field, so a good pulse examination is the most common vascular examination performed.

After performing a good neurovascular examination, reduction of the knee should be performed on the field or sideline. The reduction is normally not difficult due to the large number of torn ligaments. It is usually accomplished by pulling traction in the opposite direction of the dislocation, with a second provider stabilizing the patient by holding the femur. There is typically a palpable clunk when the joint reduces (**Fig. 4**).[11] The neurovascular examination should be repeated and documented after the successful reduction.

Posterolateral knee dislocations may be irreducible using closed reduction techniques. This occurs when the medial femoral condyle buttonholes through the medial capsule and medial collateral ligament. If initial reduction is not successful, the sports medicine provider should look for a dimple sign medially, which is frequently seen when the condyle has button holed through the capsule. No more than 2 closed reductions should be attempted because the joint is normally easily reduced. Following reduction, the leg should be splinted in approximately 10° to 15° of flexion, and the player should be immediately transported to the hospital for definitive evaluation. This is a limb-threatening injury that remains an emergency even after successful reduction of the joint. This is true even if the player has a completely normal neurovascular examination on the field. Knee dislocations represent a career-threatening injury and will require extensive surgical reconstruction and rehabilitation.

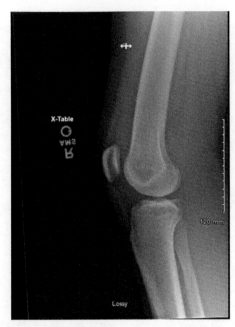

Fig. 4. Postreduction radiograph of dislocation shown in **Fig. 3**.

Patellofemoral joint (PFJ) dislocations are a far more common type of knee dislocation than tibiofemoral joint dislocations.[11] Acute PFJ dislocations can occur from a direct blow or because of an internal rotation twisting injury combined with valgus stress with a planted foot. This occurs frequently with landing from a jump classically seen in basketball or gymnastics.[11] Reduction is normally straightforward and accomplished with medial pressure on the laterally dislocated patella while gently extending the knee. PFJ dislocations do not represent an emergency but athletes usually have significant pain and swelling. They will not be able to return to play on the same day. Chronic dislocators may have minimal pain and swelling and may be able to return to play in the game. There are many recent developments in the long-term treatment of athletes following PFJ dislocations that are beyond the scope of this article. There is a trend toward surgical treatment of some first-time dislocators depending on the number of risk factors for repeat dislocations.

Hip dislocations

Hip dislocations are emergent injuries. Although uncommon, it can occur with collision sports, most frequently with football.[11] About 70% of all hip dislocations are posterior, and 90% of those injuries occur while participating in athletics. Football and rugby are the most common sports where hip dislocations occur, followed by alpine skiing and snowboarding.[11] Athletes present with severe pain, limb shortening, and hip flexion and adduction.

Initial treatment should focus on a good neurovascular examination. If this is abnormal, the athlete should be transported to the nearest trauma center immediately. If that examination in normal, the athlete should be placed supine on a back board with the hip in the most comfortable positions (usually flexion). To reduce the hip, 1 or 2 attempts should be made either on the field or in the locker room. Repeated attempts beyond that should not be performed as some dislocations are irreducible and others require sedation and muscle relaxation. There are several reductions techniques including the Allis, Stimson, Bigelow, and Whistler techniques. The team physician should familiarize him or herself with 1 or 2 of these techniques and recognize that many of them require an assistant. Early reduction is critical to help prevent osteonecrosis of the head of the femur. Hips that are reduced in less than 6 hours have a 5% risk of osteonecrosis compared with a 60% risk in hips that are dislocated for more than 6 hours.[11] Following reduction, the neurovascular examination should be repeated and documented. Common injuries in posterior hip dislocation include sciatic nerve injuries (10%–14%) and concomitant posterior wall acetabulum fractures or fractures of the femoral head, neck, or shaft. Following reduction, the athlete should be transported to a regional trauma center for evaluation and definitive treatment. Hip dislocation is usually a season ending and may be a career-ending injury.

Glenohumeral joint dislocations

Dislocations around the shoulder joint are much more common than the lower extremity dislocations discussed above but usually represent less severe injuries. About 90%[16] to 95%[11] of shoulder dislocations are anterior, with 5% posterior and less than 1% inferior.[11] It is the most commonly dislocated joint in athletes. Classically, dislocation is caused by an arm forced into abduction, external rotation, and extension. It can also occur from a direct blow from posterior but this is much less common.[11] Athletes with anterior dislocations present with severe pain with the arm slightly abducted and internally rotated. A simple practical test is to ask the athlete if they can grab the opposite shoulder. If they cannot, it is likely the shoulder is dislocated anteriorly.[11] Posterior dislocations have the arm adducted and internally rotated.

Initial treatment should include an evaluation of the patient for associated injuries. A neurovascular examination must be included and documented before any attempt at reduction. Ten percent of primary anterior shoulder dislocations have an axillary nerve neuropraxia, with 1% to 2% having a vascular injury.[16] The pathognomonic triad for injury to the axillary artery is an anterior shoulder dislocation, diminished or absent radial pulse, and a palpable axillary hematoma.[16] Other concerning physical examination signs that should prompt additional evaluation include obvious deformity of the humerus, decreased sensation, or discoloration of the extremity.[17]

Reduction of shoulder dislocations in the prehospital setting is well accepted and recommended if there are no emergent conditions requiring immediate transport.[11,16–18] Success rates for early reduction without sedation are reported to be approximately 90%, which is not significantly different than reported in hospital rates of successful reduction.[18] We recommend prompt reduction performed in the locker room to minimize distractions and spectators.[11] There are several described techniques that work well. Some require 2 people but others require only one.[11,16–18] It is wise to become familiar with more than one technique and to learn at least one reduction maneuver that can be performed by a single sports medicine provider. Following reduction, the arm should be placed into a sling for comfort. There is some debate regarding the ideal position of the arm for nonoperative treatment of shoulder dislocations. The ultimate position should be determined by whoever is going to manage the patient long-term. Return to play in the same season versus early surgical stabilization is also somewhat controversial and should be determined collaboratively by the athlete and sports medicine surgeon. In order to return to play, the patient must demonstrate near normal range of motion, little to no pain, normal strength, normal functional ability, and normal sports-specific skills.[19]

Sternoclavicular joint dislocations

A rare but important dislocation that can occur in athletics and must be treated as an emergency is a posterior sternoclavicular dislocation or fracture dislocation. It is more common in the pediatric population and frequently represents a physeal fracture dislocation.[20] Because of the proximity of major vascular structures with the risk of damage of those structures combined with potential breathing and/or swallowing difficulties, these injuries should be treated as an emergency. Patients should be carefully assessed for the Airway, Breathing and Circulation (ABCs) of trauma resuscitation. If initially stable they should be transported expeditiously to the regional trauma center. These injuries are normally reduced in the operating room with vascular surgeons available on standby. The results of open reduction and surgical fixation of this injury are generally good. However, 29% of patients in one report said the injury negatively affected their ability to participate in sports long-term.[20]

Wrist and hand dislocations

The final dislocation we will discuss in this article involves the interphalangeal joints of the fingers. Injuries to the wrist and hand account for 15% of all injuries in collision sports with 50% of these involving the fingers.[11] The most common finger dislocations involve the proximal interphalangeal joint (PIPJ). Dorsal dislocations are the most common, followed by lateral and then volar dislocations (**Fig. 5**). The small finger is the most commonly impacted digit.[16] Classically, there is hyperextension of the PIPJ from an axial load with the middle phalanx lying on the dorsal surface of the proximal phalanx with avulsion (often with a small bone fragment) of the volar plate from the base of the middle phalanx. Dislocations that involve a bone fragment that is greater than 40% of the articular surface are extremely unstable making it very difficult to maintain a closed reduction.[11]

Sideline evaluation of IPJ dislocations should include the assessment for rotational deformities, skin integrity, and neurovascular status. Following this initial evaluation, they should be reduced by applying axial traction, slightly increasing the deformity, and then sliding the digit back into place. The reduction is normally easily accomplished. Volar dislocations may be irreducible due to soft tissue interposition.[11] After successful reduction, the finger should be assessed for stability, neurovascular status, and active motion. Return to play on the same day can be considered if there is

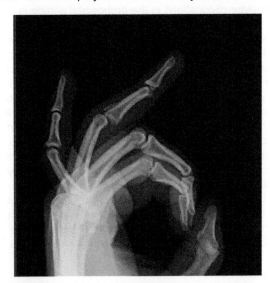

Fig. 5. Football player who sustained a volar dislocation with dorsal fracture resulting in a reduction that still has the finger volarly subluxed.

minimal pain, no neurovascular compromise, full active PIP extension, and no rotational deformity. Buddy taping or some form of functional splint should be applied before return to play.[11] Radiographs should be obtained after the game or at half time to assess the quality of reduction and any associated fractures. Dorsal and lateral PIPJ dislocations should be splinted in 20° to 30° of flexion for 2 weeks to allow for healing of the volar plate. Volar PIPJ dislocations with an associated central slip injury should be splinted in full extension for 6 weeks.[11] Joint stiffness is the most common complication but sports medicine physicians must also watch carefully for the development of swan-neck deformities from untreated volar plate injuries as well as Boutonniere deformities from central slip injuries.[11]

CLINICAL CARE POINTS

- Stabilize the injury as soon as possible to prevent further damage and reduce pain. This can help prevent further damage and reduce pain.
- Assess neurovascular status and triage accordingly.
- Rule out associated injuries such as ligament, nerve or developing compartment syndrome.
- Have a plan for safe transportation of the player before competition and be prepared to implement.
- Avoid delayed treatment by obtaining a thorough evaluation and imaging work up as needed[6]. Use clinical judgement to determine if player can return to play.

SUMMARY

Fractures and dislocations are occurring with increasing frequency in athletic competitions, including occasionally from celebrating a score or other good play.[21] Sports medicine surgeons providing game coverage must be prepared to treat these injuries on the sideline and at the venue. Many of these injuries can be treated at the venue, and in some cases, the athlete may return to play during the same contest. However, it is important to have a medical huddle before the game to review emergency plans for treatment and transport to the regional trauma center. Sports medicine physicians must be prepared to treat fractures and dislocations in athletes.

DISCLOSURE

J.P. Stannard is a board or committee member for American Orthopedic Association; is a board or committee member for AO Foundation; is a board or committee member for AO North America; is a paid consultant and receives research support from Arthrex; is a paid consultant for DePuy, A Johnson & Johnson Company; is on the editorial or governing board for the Journal of Knee Surgery; is a board or committee member for Mid-America Orthopedic Association; receives research support from the National Institutes of Health (NIAMS & NICHD); is a paid consultant for Orthopedic Designs North America; is a paid consultant for Smith & Nephew; receives publishing royalties, financial or material support from Thieme; and receives research support from U.S. Department of Defense.

REFERENCES

1. Kramer DE, Pace JL. Acute traumatic and sports-related osteochondral injury of the pediatric knee. Orthop Clin North Am 2012;43(2):227–36, vi.

2. Aitken SA, Watson BS, Wood AM, et al. Sports-related fractures in South East Scotland: an analysis of 990 fractures. J Orthop Surg Hong Kong 2014;22(3): 313–7.

3. Robertson GAJ, Wood AM. Return to Sport After Tibial Shaft Fractures: A Systematic Review. Sports Health 2016;8(4):324–30.

4. Chaturvedi A, Mann L, Cain U, et al. Acute Fractures and Dislocations of the Ankle and Foot in Children. Radiographics 2020;40(3):754–74.

5. Robertson GAJ, Wood AM, Aitken SA, et al. Epidemiology, management, and outcome of sport-related ankle fractures in a standard UK population. Foot Ankle Int 2014;35(11):1143–52.

6. British Orthopaedic Association Trauma Committee. British orthopaedic association standard for trauma (BOAST): Diagnosis & management of arterial injuries associated with extremity fractures and dislocations. Injury 2021;52(7):1667–9.

7. Vanlommel L, Vanlommel J, Bollars P, et al. Incidence and risk factors of lower leg fractures in Belgian soccer players. Injury 2013;44(12):1847–50.

8. Van den Broek M, Oussedik S. Paediatric fractures around the knee. Br J Hosp Med Lond Engl 2005 2017;78(8):453–8.

9. Bharam S, Vrahas MS, Fu FH. Knee fractures in the athlete. Orthop Clin North Am 2002;33(3):565–74.

10. Teissier V, Tresson P, Gaudric J, et al. Importance of Early Diagnosis and Care in Knee Dislocations Associated with Vascular Injuries. Ann Vasc Surg 2019;61: 238–45.

11. Schupp CM, Rand SE, Hanson TW, et al. Sideline Management of Joint Dislocations. Curr Sports Med Rep 2016;15(3):140–53.

12. Stannard JP, Lopez R, Volgas D. Soft tissue injury of the knee after tibial plateau fractures. J Knee Surg 2010;23(4):187–92.

13. Stannard JP, Schreiner AJ. Vascular Injuries following Knee Dislocation. J Knee Surg 2020;33(4):351–6.

14. Stannard JP, Sheils TM, Lopez-Ben RR, et al. Vascular injuries in knee dislocations: the role of physical examination in determining the need for arteriography. J Bone Joint Surg Am 2004;86(5):910–5.

15. Mills WJ, Barei DP, McNair P. The value of the ankle-brachial index for diagnosing arterial injury after knee dislocation: a prospective study. J Trauma 2004;56(6): 1261–5.

16. Shah R, Chhaniyara P, Wallace WA, et al. Pitch-side management of acute shoulder dislocations: a conceptual review. BMJ Open Sport Exerc Med 2016;2(1): e000116.

17. Carr JB, Chicklo B, Altchek DW, et al. On-field Management of Shoulder and Elbow Injuries in Baseball Athletes. Curr Rev Musculoskelet Med 2019;12(2): 67–71.

18. Fraser C, Pellatt R, Shirran M, et al. Early reduction of acute anterior shoulder dislocations in a ski field setting. Emerg Med Australas EMA 2022;34(3):449–51.

19. McCarty EC, Ritchie P, Gill HS, et al. Shoulder instability: return to play. Clin Sports Med 2004;23(3):335–51, vii-viii.

20. Swarup I, Cazzulino A, Williams BA, et al. Outcomes After Surgical Fixation of Posterior Sternoclavicular Physeal Fractures and Dislocations in Children. J Pediatr Orthop 2021;41(1):11–6.

21. Momaya A, Read C, Estes R. When celebrations go wrong: a case series of injuries after celebrating in sports. J Sports Med Phys Fitness 2017;57(3):267–71.

Acute Compartment Syndrome in the Athlete

Omar Farah, BS[a], Ghassan Farah, MD[b], Salma Mumuni, MD[b], Elan Volchenko, MD[b], Mark R. Hutchinson, MD[b,*]

KEYWORDS

- Acute compartment syndrome • Fasciotomy • Sports • Sideline management
- Tibial fracture

KEY POINTS

- Early recognition of acute compartment syndrome is critical for optimal treatment and recovery.
- Intracompartment pressure monitoring is helpful to confirm diagnosis but not required to perform surgical intervention in obvious cases.
- Once diagnosis is made, the treatment of acute compartment syndrome is emergent surgical decompressive fasciotomy.
- Protective measures including removing compressive dressings, spitting casts, stabilization of fractures, maintaining the extremity at the level of the heart, foot pumps, and oxygen therapy may reduce the risk of conversion to acute compartment syndrome in high risk patients.

INTRODUCTION/HISTORY/DEFINITIONS/BACKGROUND

Compartment syndrome is a painful condition that results from increased pressure within a muscle compartment. It can be further divided into acute compartment syndrome (ACS) and chronic compartment syndrome. Although the pathophysiology underlying acute and chronic compartment syndrome is similar, they have differing etiologies, presentations, and complications. ACS represents one of the few surgical emergencies in orthopedic surgery, thus necessitating prompt diagnosis to ensure timely and adequate management.[1]

History

One of the earliest definitive acknowledgments of ACS and its consequences was made by the German doctor, Volkmann, in 1881. Volkmann described what is now known as a "Volkmann's contracture": a deformity of the hand, fingers, or wrist caused

[a] Columbia University Vagelos College of Physicians and Surgeons; [b] Department of Orthopaedic Surgery, University of Illinois, Chicago, USA
* Corresponding author. 835 South Wolcott, 270 MSB, Chicago, IL 60612, USA
E-mail address: mhutch@uic.edu

Clin Sports Med 42 (2023) 525–538
https://doi.org/10.1016/j.csm.2023.02.013
0278-5919/23/© 2023 Elsevier Inc. All rights reserved.

by ischemic injury to the forearm secondary to ACS.[2] In 1888, Petersen provided the earliest report of ACS management.[3] He believed that the condition resulted from arterial occlusion and inflammation within the compartment and reported that decompression of the forearm led to alleviation of some symptoms and return of nerve function.[4] This gave way to more studies on the etiology and management of ACS, including Murphy's revelation in 1914 that the cause of ACS was due to hemorrhage within the compartment, specifically secondary to bone fracture.[4] Murphy was the first to suggest fasciotomy as management of ACS.

Throughout the 1900s, studies regarding the management of ACS accumulated. Although there was a general consensus that fasciotomy was the treatment of choice and provided the best outcomes for ACS patients, the preferred techniques of the procedure remained controversial.[4] Today, debate continues surrounding the diagnosis of compartment syndrome and the optimal surgical techniques.

Pathophysiology

A compartment is a well-defined region within a limb that contains a set of muscles, vasculature, and nerves.[5] Compartments are separated from one another by thick fascia that is resistant to stretch or expansion.[5] ACS occurs when an injury to the limb leads to an appreciable increase in intracompartmental pressure (ICP).[6] The initial injury can be of varying etiologies, including traumatic and hemorrhagic, among others. The increase in pressure is enough to compress the thin-walled venules within the compartment, leading to a decrease in drainage of the compartment, further increasing the hydrostatic compartment pressure.[3] A vicious cycle of rapidly increasing compartment pressure begins which eventually causes the pressure to reach a level that can compress the thicker-walled arteries and arterioles within the compartment.[7] The result is decreased perfusion pressure, with subsequent ischemia to muscles and nerves. Prolonged ischemia may result in tissue necrosis and its complications.

In contrast, chronic compartment syndrome, or chronic exertional compartment syndrome (CECS), occurs without acute injury or insult to the limb. Rather, CECS is secondary to increased muscle perfusion and edema that occurs during exertional activities.[8] This similarly raises ICP which leads to reduced venous return and ischemic pain. However, permanent damage is rare in CECS and symptoms typically resolve completely during a period of rest, resuming with repeated onset of exertional activity.[8] Distinguishing between acute and CECS is critical for the covering physician, as only one necessitates emergent, invasive treatment.

Symptoms and Signs

The initial presenting symptom of ACS is typically pain that is out of proportion to the examination. In such scenarios, the evaluating physician must maintain a high index of suspicion in the athlete lacking any other indicators of compartment syndrome. As the ICP rises, more symptoms and signs become present and are commonly categorized into the "6 Ps": passive pain (disproportionate to the injury or with passive stretch of the affected muscle), paresthesia, pallor, paralysis, pulselessness, and poikilothermia (difference in temperature between limbs with the affected limb being cooler).[9,10] However, these "classic" signs and symptoms are less useful in the acute evaluation of the injured athlete as they often present in delayed fashion, indicative that the extent of the injury has likely become irreversible.

Patients presenting with CECS also present with pain out of proportion to the examination. They can also experience cramping, tightness, loss of strength, and paresthesias.[8,11] The symptoms of CECS completely resolve during rest and between periods of exertional activity, which differentiates it from ACS. The clinician must be alert that it is possible for a CECS to convert to an ACS if the load challenge persists and no rest and relaxation occurs.

In Sports

Although the incidence and prevalence of CECS in sports are much higher than ACS, CECS is not a medical emergency.[8,11] Thus, this article focuses strictly on ACS in sports as to remain in line with the title of this issue, "On Field Emergencies."

PREVALENCE/INCIDENCE

The incidence of ACS in the Western world is about 3.1 per 100,000 individuals per year, with men being at a 10 times higher risk than women.[12] Men younger than 29 year old are at the highest risk for ACS, which is thought to be due to increased muscle bulk, stronger fascial structures, and a greater incidence of high-energy injuries.[12-14] Greater than two-thirds of ACS cases are secondary to fractures, and the three most common fractures leading to ACS are segmental tibia fractures (48% risk of ACS), bicondylar tibial plateau fractures (18% risk of ACS), and medial knee fracture-dislocations (53% risk of ACS).[15,16] Radius and ulna fractures are also associated with ACS, albeit, less frequently.[3] Although typically associated with fractures, ACS can also develop secondary to blunt soft tissue injury, crush injury, burns, and ballistic trauma.[3,15,17] Research has demonstrated that soft tissue injury may account for nearly 25% of ACS cases.[16] Although exceedingly rare, ACS may present with no history of preceding injury.

Regarding sporting events and athletics, tibia fractures are the most common cause of ACS.[14,15] As high as 55% of tibial fractures in soccer and 27% of tibial fractures in American football have been reported to result in ACS.[15,18] The risk of ACS increases with each additional presenting symptom of the condition, from approximately 25% when one symptom is present, to 68% when two symptoms are present, and to 93% when three or more symptoms are present.[15]

Although there is a common perception that ACS occurs exclusively in closed fractures, several studies have shown a lack of association between development of ACS and whether a diaphyseal fracture was open or closed.[10,16,19] This is likely due to the fact that minor fascial tears in some open fractures are not sufficient to decompress a muscular compartment.

EVALUATION

Evaluation of the patient in an acute setting is an integral aspect in the management of ACS. Prompt recognition of this pathology is necessary to avoid the significant morbidities associated with it, such as long-term neurovascular deficits, loss of limb, rhabdomyolysis, renal failure, and death.[17,20] Awareness of clinical scenarios in which the prevalence of ACS is increased can help clue clinicians into the patients who are at increased risk.

The earliest symptom of ACS is pain, which is frequently perceived to be out of proportion to the injury.[21] The pain is often described as severe, deep, burning, and worsened with passive stretch of the affected compartment musculature.[17,22] Pain with passive stretch has been reported to have a sensitivity of 97% and a negative predictive value of 98% in the diagnosis of ACS.[17] Patients with ACS typically have tenderness to palpation, tenseness or firmness of the affected compartment, and swelling to the affected area.[17,21] Delayed symptoms of ACS result from prolonged nerve ischemia and include paresthesias, sensory deficits, and motor weakness.[15,17,21] Because of the possible sensory loss in ACS, pain may be absent in later stages.[17] The evaluating physician must remain cognizant that signs and symptoms of ACS are inherently subjective and nonspecific. Although the combination of pain with passive stretch, paresthesias, and pain at rest is associated with 93% sensitivity in the diagnosis of ACS and 98% sensitivity when combined with paresis, diagnosis is ideally made before the onset of this delayed presentation.[17,21]

The anterior compartment of the leg is the most common location of ACS, likely due to the high incidence of tibial fractures and the compartment's inability to accommodate volume changes.[17] The anterior compartment of the leg may be palpated anterolaterally between the tibia and fibula and passively stretched with plantarflexion of the ankle. The superficial and deep posterior compartments of the leg may also be involved, though less commonly than the anterior compartment. Examination of these compartments involves posterior palpation and passive stretching with dorsiflexion of the ankle. The deep posterior compartment of the lower extremity may also be passively stretched with eversion of the foot. Of note, the deep posterior compartment is often difficult to palpate given the overlying gastroc-soleus complex and appreciable swelling or tenseness of the compartment may be impossible to evaluate at a sporting event. If necessary, further evaluation may include ICP measurements (described below). The lateral compartment of the lower extremity is palpated directly lateral to the fibula and is passively stretched with dorsiflexion of the ankle and inversion of the foot. ACS can also develop in the thigh, with the anterior compartment most frequently involved.[17] The anterior compartment of the thigh is passively stretched with knee flexion. Conversely, the posterior compartment of the thigh is passively stretched with knee extension. In the forearm, the anterior compartment is palpated in the volar forearm and passively stretched with finger and wrist extension. The posterior compartment is palpated dorsally at the forearm and is passively stretched with finger and wrist flexion. The mobile wad compartment of the forearm is difficult to assess in isolation, as the musculature contained in the compartment has overlap in action and passive stretch with the anterior and posterior compartments. Regarding ACS in the hand, intrinsic muscles can be evaluated with passive abduction and adduction of the digits with the metacarpophalangeal (MCP) joints in extension and the proximal interphalangeal (PIP) joints in flexion. The adductor compartment of the hand is stretched with passive palmar abduction of the thumb. The thenar muscles are stretched by abduction and extension of the thumb, and the hypothenar muscles are stretched by abduction and extension of the little finger.[23,24] ACS of the foot can be evaluated using passive movement of the toes; however, it is notoriously difficult to distinguish between compartments. A summary of clinical signs associated with compartment syndrome is presented in **Table 1**.

If available, pulse oximetry can be used to quickly assess limb perfusion. Critically, however, normal blood oxygen reading *does not* rule out ACS.[1,16,17,21]

APPROACH/GUIDELINES

There is currently no physical examination finding or diagnostic test that has 100% specificity and sensitivity for ACS. Thus, medical providers need to use a combination of the symptoms, risk factors, clinical time course, and diagnostics tests to aid them with the diagnosis of ACS.[3]

In 2019, the American Academy of Orthopedic Surgeons (AAOS) created the Clinical Practice Guideline (CPG) for the Management of ACS to provide orthopedic surgeons and other providers with a guide for initial assessment and treatment of patients at risk

Table 1
Clinical signs associated with each compartment syndrome[33]

Compartment	Signs
Thigh	
Anterior	Pain with passive knee flexion Numbness of the medial leg/foot Weakness in knee extension
Posterior	Pain with passive knee extension Sensory changes rare Weakness in knee flexion
Adductor	Pain on passive hip abduction Sensory changes rare Weakness in hip adduction
Leg	
Anterior	Pain with passive flexion of ankle and toes Numbness in the first webspace Weakness in ankle and toe extension
Lateral	Pain with passive foot inversion Numbness of the dorsal foot Weakness in eversion
Superficial posterior	Pain with passive ankle extension Numbness of the dorsal lateral foot Weakness in plantarflexion
Deep posterior	Pain with passive ankle and toe extension Pain with foot eversion Numbness of the sole of the foot Weakness in toe and ankle flexion Weakness in foot inversion
Foot	
All compartments (nonspecific)	Pain in the foot with passive toe motion Increased pain and swelling of the foot
Arm	
Anterior	Pain with passive elbow extension Numbness in an ulnar/median distribution Numbness in the volar/lateral distal forearm Weakness in elbow flexion Weakness in median/ulnar motor function
Posterior	Pain with passive elbow flexion Numbness in an ulnar/radial distribution Weakness in elbow extension Weakness in radial/ulnar motor
Forearm	
Volar	Pain with passive wrist and finger extension Numbness in a median/ulnar distribution Weakness in wrist and finger flexion Weakness in hand median/ulnar motor function
Dorsal	Pain with passive wrist and finger flexion Weakness in wrist and finger flexion
Mobile wad	Pain with passive wrist and elbow extension Weakness in wrist extension and elbow flexion

(continued on next page)

Table 1 (continued)	
Compartment	**Signs**
Hand	
Interosseous	Pain with passive abduction of digits in MCP extension and PIP flexion
Thenar	Pain with passive abduction and extension of the thumb
Hypothenar	Pain with passive abduction and extension of the small finger

of compartment syndrome based on evidence-based principles from over 3,600 abstracts and more than 480 full-text articles.[25,26] The AAOS CPG of ACS recommended the use of frequent serial examinations for making any definitive diagnosis. It is also recommended having the same surgeon perform the serial assessments and that the findings should be clearly documented.[3]

Although compartment syndrome is generally considered a clinical diagnosis, measuring ICPs is a well-established method for diagnosing ACS, especially in unconscious/intubated patients where most of the clinical findings cannot be elicited. McQueen and colleagues reported in a retrospective study that intracompartment pressure monitoring in suspected ACS had a sensitivity of 93%, an estimated specificity of 98%, an estimated positive predictive value of 93%, and an estimated negative predictive value of 99%.[27] However, there is some variation in the literature on pressure measurement method, timing, and thresholds.[27,28]

Various techniques for measuring ICP include a hand-held monitor for single pressure readings, Stryker needle with side portal (**Fig. 1**), and regular needle with arterial line setup.[3] A study by Heckman and colleagues found that in the setting of a fracture, compartment pressures were found to be different at various locations within compartments in relation to the injury site. Therefore, they suggested that pressure can be measured in different sites in all compartments but within 5 cm of the fracture site.[29]

There is still little consensus among authors on what values of compartment pressures should be considered as the threshold for surgical decompressive fasciotomy. Mubarak and colleagues used an absolute value of 45 mm Hg for diagnosis of ACS and indication for fasciotomy, whereas 30 mm Hg was used by Matsen and colleagues.[28,30] Gelberman and colleagues also recommended compartment fasciotomies for compartment pressures greater than 30 mm Hg.[31] Whiteside and colleagues were the first authors to suggest the importance of the difference between the diastolic blood pressure and ICP or ΔP. They concluded that a ΔP less than 30 mm Hg was a safe threshold for decompression in ACS.[32] It is important to note that the AAOS CPG of ACS recommends against using a single pressure value alone for diagnosing compartment syndrome as this may lead to unnecessary surgery. ICPs should be used in addition to clinical suspicion and physical examination findings to aid in diagnosis.[25]

SURGICAL TECHNIQUES
Intro to Fasciotomy

The current standard of care for treatment of ACS is surgical decompressive fasciotomy.[33] Other preliminary measures may be taken before surgical intervention to

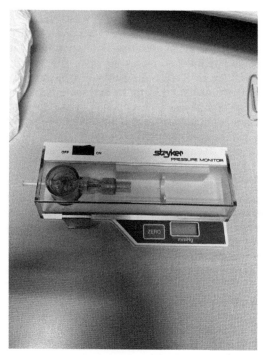

Fig. 1. STIC (formally Stryker) pressure monitor unit.

reduce ICP. These include removal of any compressive dressings, splitting and spreading of casts or splints, and temporary reduction and stabilization of associated fractures or dislocations.[34] The affected limb should not be elevated above the level of the heart, as this may result in decreased extremity perfusion and exacerbation of muscle ischemia.[35] Oxygen therapy should be initiated and any hemodynamic instability reversed to optimally perfuse the affected extremity tissue.[33]

Indications for Fasciotomy

As mentioned above, indications for surgical decompressive fasciotomy are inconsistent in the literature. Some assert ACS is a clinical diagnosis. Others rely on ICP measurements, citing the poor sensitivity of clinical examination with high false-negative rates, or missed diagnoses.[33] Regardless of method used, once a diagnosis is made, emergent fasciotomy is indicated to release the fascial compartment and restore perfusion to the tissue.[33] Delayed treatment is commonly implicated in litigations against clinicians, especially orthopedic surgeons, for compartment syndrome complications, which may include infection, muscle weakness, limb paralysis, ischemic contractures, and limb amputation.[33]

Common Surgical Approach

The principle of surgical fasciotomy is to fully decompress the affected compartment. Limited approaches have no role in fasciotomy for ACS. Rather, lengthy skin incisions should be made traversing the entire length of the compartment that allows decompression of both the skin and fascia which may contribute to the restrictive anatomy. This allows adequate visualization of all muscles within the compartment and thorough debridement of nonviable tissue.[33]

Compartment Syndrome of the Thigh

The thigh is divided into three compartments: anterior, posterior, and medial. The anterior compartment contains the quadriceps femoris muscles (vastus lateralis, vastus medialis, vastus intermedius, rectus femoris), sartorius, and femoral nerve. The posterior compartment contains the hamstring muscles and sciatic nerve. The medial compartment contains the adductor muscles and obturator nerve.[33]

Approach to the thigh compartments is generally straightforward. A lateral incision may be used to access both the anterior and posterior compartments. Although less commonly affected, the medial (adductor) compartment may be accessed through a separate medial incision if deemed necessary.[33,36]

Compartment Syndrome of the Leg

The leg is divided into four compartments: anterior, lateral, superficial posterior, and deep posterior. The anterior compartment, the most commonly involved in ACS, contains the tibialis anterior, extensor hallucis longus, extensor digitorum longus, peroneus tertius, and deep peroneal nerve. The lateral compartment contains the peroneus brevis and longus and the superficial peroneal nerve. The posterior compartment is divided into superficial and deep components, separated by an intermuscular septum. The superficial posterior compartment contains the gastrocnemius–soleus complex and plantaris muscle. The deep posterior compartment contains the tibial posterior, flexor hallucis longus, flexor digitorum longus, and tibial nerve.[33]

All four compartments of the leg should be released, most commonly through a dual-incision approach.[37] The lateral and anterior compartments are accessed through a laterally-based incision. Care must be taken to avoid damage to the superficial peroneal nerve, especially within the distal third of the leg as it pierces the fascia to become subcutaneous. A separate medial incision is made 2 cm posterior to the medial subcutaneous border of the tibia. Skin retraction allows direct access to the superficial posterior compartment. Retraction of the superficial posterior compartment allows access to the deep posterior compartment.[33] Conversely, a single lateral incision may also be used.[38] Anterior retraction of the lateral compartment allows access to the posterior compartments. This approach is more technically challenging, especially in obtaining access to the deep posterior compartment. However, both approaches have demonstrated efficacy in reducing ICPs when performed appropriately.[33,39]

Compartment Syndrome of the Foot

The foot is divided into nine compartments: medial, lateral, deep (calcaneal) central, superficial central, adductor hallucis, and four interosseous compartments. High index of suspicion is required in the setting of severe swelling of the foot; however, distinguishing between foot compartments is difficult.[33,40]

Two dorsal incisions overlying the second and fourth metatarsals allow access to the four interosseous compartments, the central compartments, and the medial and lateral compartments (around the deep surfaces of the first and fifth metatarsals, respectively). In the setting of calcaneus fractures, a separate medial incision may be required to adequately decompress the deep calcaneal compartment.[33,41]

Compartment Syndrome of the Arm

The arm is divided into two compartments. The anterior compartment contains the brachialis, biceps brachii, coracobrachialis, median nerve, ulnar nerve (proximally), musculocutaneous nerve, lateral cutaneous nerve, antebrachial nerve, and radial nerve (distally). The posterior compartment contains the triceps brachii, radial nerve, and ulnar nerve (distally).[33] Separate anterior and posterior incisions allow direct and easy access for decompressive fasciotomy of the arm.[33]

Compartment Syndrome of the Forearm

The forearm is divided into three compartments. The volar compartment includes the wrist and finger flexors, pronator teres, pronator quadratus, median nerve, and ulnar nerve. The dorsal aspect of the forearm is subdivided into two separate compartments. The dorsal compartment includes the extensor digitorum communis, extensor pollicis longus, abductor pollicis longus, and extensor carpi ulnaris. The "mobile wad" contains the brachioradialis, extensor carpi radialis brevis, and extensor carpi radialis longus.

The forearm may normally be adequately decompressed through a single volar incision.[42] The incision extends from the biceps tendon proximally toward the wrist distally, allowing concurrent decompression of the carpal tunnel. In some cases, persistently elevated pressures indicate the need for associated decompression of the dorsal compartment, which can be directly accessed through a longitudinal dorsal incision.[33]

Compartment Syndrome of the Hand

The hand is divided into 10 compartments: thenar, hypothenar, three volar interosseous, four dorsal interosseous, and adductor pollicis compartments.[33] Adequate decompression may be achieved through two dorsal incisions allowing access to the interosseous compartments. Occasionally, separate volar-based decompressions of the thenar and hypothenar compartments are required.[33]

Fasciotomy Wound Closure and Postoperative Care

Primary closure of fasciotomy wounds should be avoided, as this may result in recurrence of increased ICPs.[33,43] Instead, the wounds should be left open and dressed appropriately. Oftentimes, a "second look" procedure is indicated to ensure viability of tissue at approximately the 48-hour mark. In the absence of necrosis, a delayed primary closure may be performed at this point. Wounds may be difficult to approximate, in which case other techniques may be used, including dermatotraction, split thickness skin grafting, and negative pressure wound vac therapy. Dermatotraction may be complicated by in peri-incisional wound necrosis, whereas split thickness skin grafting involves donor site morbidity.[44,45]

CLINICAL OUTCOMES

Compartment syndrome results in reduced perfusion to extremity tissues. The resultant ischemia is intuitively correlated with the length of time of hypoperfusion, making early recognition and treatment a crucial aspect of management of athletes at risk. The concept of hypoperfusion should account for a range of either complete circulation cutoff or simply gradually progressive diminished flow. The latter may account for "some" perfusion that extends the vitality of the challenged tissues. In general, outcomes following compartment syndrome may be favorable in the setting of timely diagnosis and decompression.[33,46] Factors potentially associated with poor outcomes include severe crush injuries, arterial injuries, and associated fractures.[31,47]

Timing of Diagnosis and Treatment

The sections above detail the critical aspects for early diagnosis of compartment syndrome in the acutely injured athlete. These include knowledge of commonly associated mechanisms and presentations, sound clinical examination, and use of ICP measurements when indicated. In the obtunded patient, a high index of suspicion is necessary. A missed or delayed diagnosis may have devastating consequences for the patient. Studies have cited delay in diagnosis as the primary reason for failure in management of ACS.[33,48]

For example, ACS of the thigh is a rare entity and thus is often subject to missed or late diagnosis. Mithoefer and colleagues demonstrated high rates of morbidity associated with ACS of the thigh and a correlation with prolonged intervals to decompression and presence of muscle necrosis at time of decompression.[47] Specifically, ischemia time of more than 6 hours may result in an array of complications, including functional disability, sensory loss, infection, and poor associated fracture healing.[33,49] Finkelstein and colleagues demonstrated poor outcomes with delayed fasciotomy more than 35 hours following established lower limb compartment syndrome. Complications included multisystem organ failure, limb amputation, and infection.[50]

Complications

Volkmann contractures

With prolonged hypoperfusion, irreversible muscle necrosis occurs within the compartment. Subsequent contractures may develop further limited functionality of the affected limb.[46]

In the forearm, varying degrees of contracture may occur, with the most common deformity including elbow flexion, forearm protonation, wrist flexion, thumb adduction, MCP joint extension, and interphalangeal joint flexion. Treatments involve lysis of adhesions, debridement of necrotic tissue, neurolysis, tenolysis, tendon transfers, and free muscle transfers. Yet, return of normal functionality is rare.[46]

The most common deformity following foot compartment syndrome is claw toe, which develops due to intrinsic–extrinsic muscle imbalance. Other deformities include hammer toes and cavus with resultant ulcerations.[51]

Infection

Postoperative infection following decompressive fasciotomy represents a common complication that may result in devastating complications, including amputation and death. Studies have cited an incidence of up to 30% for post-fasciotomy surgical site infections. Merchan and colleagues demonstrated that time to closure following fasciotomy, specifically more than 4 to 5 days postoperatively, was associated with an increased risk of infection. As mentioned above, immediate primary closure following fasciotomy is not recommended. Delayed primary closure may be difficult given associated swelling, necessitating the use of dermatotraction techniques and skin grafting.[52]

Treatment in Cases of Late Diagnosis

Controversy exists regarding the treatment of a missed or delayed compartment syndrome diagnosis. Oftentimes, the intracompartmental muscles have already undergone necrosis, without potential for recovery of function. In these cases, decompressive fasciotomy has little utility to justify its associated surgical morbidity. Finkelstein and colleagues demonstrated high morbidity with delayed fasciotomy and recommended reconsideration of traditional fasciotomy in diagnoses delayed more than 8 to 10 hours.[50] In the absence of muscle function, surgical intervention is generally avoided.[53] Instead, treatment of systemic complications, including myoglobinuria, and splinting to prevent common contractures is indicated.[46,53] On the other hand, there are cases in which viable muscle exists among largely necrotic tissue. In the setting of demonstrable muscle function and persistently elevated compartment pressures, decompressive fasciotomy is indicated to salvage residual limb functionality.[33,53]

DISCUSSION

Surgical decompressive fasciotomy is an effective treatment for ACS. As discussed thoroughly above, timely intervention to reduce ICPs is strongly correlated to the reduction of long term morbidity. Although the completeness of vascular flow and hypoperfusion must be taken into account, the contrary also holds true, with delayed diagnosis of compartment syndrome being the single most important influence on outcomes. For this reason, much of current research is aimed at optimizing the process of compartment syndrome diagnosis.[54]

The current gold standard for diagnosis of ACS remains clinical. Yet, recent research has demonstrated high sensitivity and specificity of ICP monitoring, calling into question the long-held belief that compartment syndrome is a clinical diagnosis.[33] ICP monitoring is an invasive procedure, which likely partially contributes to hesitancy in its use. Clinicians of all specialties need to be educated regarding the simplicity and effectiveness of currently available devices to optimize their use. Currently, noninvasive modalities for monitoring tissue perfusion are also under study. The addition of ubiquitous guidelines for efficient and accurate diagnosis of ACS in all units caring for trauma patients may also reduce the time to fasciotomy.

The risk factors for compartment syndrome have been studied extensively. These include certain mechanisms of injury (ie, high energy, crush) and specific fractures (ie, tibial shaft). Nevertheless, the current methods for preventing compartment syndrome are limited and include icing, elevation of the affected extremity, and skeletal stabilization. Future interventions may additionally address fluid shifts on a systemic level, preventing the accumulation of fluid within an affected compartment, or involve the administration of antioxidants to prevent toxic injury to muscle.[33,55–57]

SUMMARY

In sports, ACS is typically a result of lower limb fracture, leading to high ICPs and pain out of proportion to the physical examination in the affected limb. The prompt diagnosis of acute compartment syndrome is the critical to a successful outcome. High intra-compartment pressures that persist for 6 to 8 hours are likely to result in irreversible damage to muscles and nerves. The goal of treatment of ACS is to reduce ICP through decompressive fasciotomy to facilitate reperfusion of ischemic tissue. Improved awareness and early recognition followed by expedited intervention will lead to reduced complications and improved long-term functional outcomes. A delay in diagnosis and treatment can lead to significant complications such as permanent sensory and motor deficits, contractures, infection and in extreme cases, amputation of the limb or death.

CLINICS CARE POINTS

- In sports, acute compartment syndrome is most commonly secondary to tibial fracture. Awareness of other clinical scenarios in which the prevalence of acute compartment syndrome is increased may help clue clinicians into the athletes who are at increased risk.

- Acute compartment syndrome has historically been a clinical diagnosis. However, intracompartmental pressure monitoring is increasing in popularity, with possibly superior diagnostic accuracy.
- Prompt recognition of this pathology is necessary to avoid the significant associated morbidities. The absence of the "6 Ps" does not rule out compartment syndrome. High index of suspicion is necessary to early diagnosis, especially in cases of uncontrolled pain.
- Once diagnosis has been made, treatment of acute compartment syndrome is through emergent and thorough surgical decompressive fasciotomy.
- Fasciotomy should involve lengthy incisions covering the entire compartment and allowing thorough and complete decompression. The primary closure of skin is not recommended.
- Delayed treatment may result in infection, sensory deficit, limb weakness/paralysis, ischemic contractures, and limb amputation.

DISCLOSURE

The authors declare that they have no relevant material or financial interests associated with the contents of this chapter.

REFERENCES

1. Via AG, Oliva F, Spoliti M, et al. Acute compartment syndrome. Muscles Ligaments Tendons J 2015;5(1):18–22.
2. R V. Die ischaemischen muskellahmungen und kontrakturen. Centralblat fur hirurgie 1881;8:801–3.
3. Raza H, Mahapatra A. Acute compartment syndrome in orthopedics: causes, diagnosis, and management. Advances in Orthopedics 2015;2015:e543412.
4. Rorabeck C. The treatment of compartment syndromes of the leg. J Bone Jt Surg Br Vol 1984;66-B(1):93–7.
5. Compartment syndrome - orthoInfo - AAOS. Available at: https://www.orthoinfo.org/en/diseases–conditions/compartment-syndrome/. Accessed November 18, 2022.
6. Tiwari A, Haq AI, Myint F, et al. Acute compartment syndromes. BJS (British Journal of Surgery) 2002;89(4):397–412.
7. Lagerstrom CF, Reed RL, Rowlands BJ, et al. Early fasciotomy for acute clinically evident posttraumatic compartment syndrome. Am J Surg 1989;158(1):36–9.
8. Liu B, Barrazueta G, Ruchelsman DE. Chronic exertional compartment syndrome in athletes. J Hand Surg 2017;42(11):917–23.
9. Cohen M, Garfin, Hargens A, et al. Acute compartment syndrome. effect of dermotomy on fascial decompression in the leg. J Bone Jt Surg Br Vol 1991;73-B(2):287–90.
10. Köstler W, Strohm PC, Südkamp NP. Acute compartment syndrome of the limb. Injury 2005;36(8):992–8.
11. Vajapey S, Miller TL. Evaluation, diagnosis, and treatment of chronic exertional compartment syndrome: a review of current literature. Physician Sportsmed 2017;45(4):391–8.
12. McQueen MM, Gaston P, Court-Brown CM. Acute compartment syndrome. J Bone Jt Surg Br Vol 2000;82-B(2):200–3.
13. Lollo L, Grabinsky A. Clinical and functional outcomes of acute lower extremity compartment syndrome at a Major Trauma Hospital. Int J Crit Illn Inj Sci 2016; 6(3):133–42.

14. McQueen MM, Duckworth AD, Aitken SA, et al. Predictors of compartment syndrome after tibial fracture. J Orthop Trauma 2015;29(10):451–5.
15. Schmidt AH. Acute compartment syndrome. Injury 2017;48:S22–5.
16. Duckworth AD, McQueen MM. The diagnosis of acute compartment syndrome: a critical analysis review. JBJS Reviews 2017;5(12):e1.
17. Long B, Koyfman A, Gottlieb M. Evaluation and management of acute compartment syndrome in the emergency department. J Emerg Med 2019;56(4):386–97.
18. Wind TC, Saunders SM, Barfield WR, et al. Compartment syndrome after low-energy tibia fractures sustained during athletic competition. J Orthop Trauma 2012;26(1):33–6.
19. Park S, Ahn J, Gee AO, et al. Compartment syndrome in tibial fractures. J Orthop Trauma 2009;23(7):514–8.
20. Schwartz JT, Brumback RJ, Lakatos R, et al. Acute compartment syndrome of the thigh. a spectrum of injury. J Bone Joint Surg Am 1989;71(3):392–400.
21. Ulmer T. The clinical diagnosis of compartment syndrome of the lower leg: are clinical findings predictive of the disorder? J Orthop Trauma 2002;16(8):572–7.
22. Donaldson J, Haddad B, Khan WS. The pathophysiology, diagnosis and current management of acute compartment syndrome. Open Orthop J 2014;8:185–93.
23. Kistler JM, Ilyas AM, Thoder JJ. Forearm compartment syndrome: evaluation and management. Hand Clin 2018;34(1):53–60.
24. Harvey EJ, Sanders DW, Shuler MS, et al. What's new in acute compartment syndrome? J Orthop Trauma 2012;26(12):699–702.
25. Osborn PM, Schmidt AH. Diagnosis and management of acute compartment syndrome. J Am Acad Orthop Surg 2021;29(5):183–8.
26. Coe MP, Osborn CPM, Schmidt AH. AAOS clinical practice guideline: management of acute compartment syndrome. J Am Acad Orthop Surg 2021;29(1):e1.
27. McQueen MM, Duckworth AD, Aitken SA, et al. The estimated sensitivity and specificity of compartment pressure monitoring for acute compartment syndrome. JBJS 2013;95(8):673–7.
28. Mubarak S, Pedowitz R, Hargens A. Compartment syndromes. Curr Orthop 1989; 3:36–40.
29. Heckman MM, Whitesides TE, Grewe SR, et al. Compartment pressure in association with closed tibial fractures. The relationship between tissue pressure, compartment, and the distance from the site of the fracture. J Bone Joint Surg Am 1994;76(9):1285–92.
30. Matseniii FA, Winquist RA, Krugmire RB. Diagnosis and Managementof Compartmental Syndromes. JBJS 1980;62(2):286–91.
31. Gelberman RH, Garfin SR, Hergenroeder PT, et al. Compartment syndromes of the forearm: diagnosis and treatment. Clin Orthop Relat Res 1981;161:252–61.
32. Whitesides TE, Haney TC, Morimoto K, et al. Tissue pressure measurements as a determinant for the need of fasciotomy. Clin Orthop Relat Res 1975;113:43–51.
33. Court-Brown C, Heckman JD, McKee M, et al. Rockwood and green's fractures in adults. Philadelphia, PA: Lippincott Williams & Wilkins; 2014.
34. Garfin SR, Mubarak SJ, Evans KL, et al. Quantification of intracompartmental pressure and volume under plaster casts. J Bone Joint Surg Am 1981;63(3): 449–53.
35. Matsen F, Wyss CR, Krugmire RB, et al. The effects of limb elevation and dependency on local arteriovenous gradients in normal human limbs with particular reference to limbs with increased tissue pressure. Clin Orthop Relat Res 1980; 150:187–95.

36. Tarlow SD, Achterman CA, Hayhurst J, et al. Acute compartment syndrome in the thigh complicating fracture of the femur. A report of three cases. JBJS 1986; 68(9):1439–43.
37. Mubarak S, OWEN C. Double-incision fasciotomy of the leg for decompression in compartment syndromes. J Bone Jt Surg Am Vol 1977;59:184–7.
38. Cooper GG. A method of single-incision, four compartment fasciotomy of the leg. Eur J Vasc Surg 1992;6(6):659–61.
39. Vitale GC, Richardson JD, George SM, et al. Fasciotomy for severe, blunt and penetrating trauma of the extremity. Surg Gynecol Obstet 1988;166(5):397–401.
40. Manoli A, Weber TG. Fasciotomy of the foot: an anatomical study with special reference to release of the calcaneal compartment. Foot Ankle 1990;10(5):267–75.
41. Myerson M, Manoli A. Compartment syndromes of the foot after calcaneal fractures. Clin Orthop Relat Res 1993;290:142–50.
42. Duckworth AD, Mitchell SE, Molyneux SG, et al. Acute compartment syndrome of the forearm. JBJS 2012;94(10):e63.
43. Havig MT, Leversedge FJ, Seiler JG. Forearm compartment pressures: an in vitro analysis of open and endoscopic assisted fasciotomy. J Hand Surg 1999;24(6): 1289–97.
44. Fitzgerald A, Wilson Y, Quaba A, et al. Long-term sequelae of fasciotomy wounds. Br J Plast Surg 2000;53(8):690–3.
45. Janzing HMJ, Broos PLO. Dermatotraction: an effective technique for the closure of fasciotomy wounds: a preliminary report of fifteen patients. J Orthop Trauma 2001;15(6):438–41.
46. Prasarn ML, Ouellette EA. Acute Compartment Syndrome of the Upper Extremity. J Am Acad Orthop Surg 2011;19(1):49–58.
47. Mithoefer K, Lhowe DW, Vrahas MS, et al. Functional outcome after acute compartment syndrome of the thigh. JBJS 2006;88(4):729–37.
48. Sheridan GW, Matsen FA. Fasciotomy in the treatment of the acute compartment syndrome. J Bone Joint Surg Am 1976;58(1):112–5.
49. Court-brown C, McQueen M. Compartment syndrome delays tibial union. Acta Orthop Scand 1987;58(3):249–52.
50. Finkelstein JA, Hunter GA, Hu RW. Lower limb compartment syndrome: course after delayed fasciotomy. J Trauma Acute Care Surg 1996;40(3):342–4.
51. Dodd A, Le I. Foot compartment syndrome: diagnosis and management. J Am Acad Orthop Surg 2013;21(11):657–64.
52. Merchan N, Ingalls B, Garcia J, et al. Factors associated with surgical site infections after fasciotomy in patients with compartment syndrome. J Am Acad Orthop Surg Glob Res Rev 2022;6(2):e22.00002.
53. Olson SA, Glasgow RR. Acute compartment syndrome in lower extremity musculoskeletal trauma. J Am Acad Orthop Surg 2005;13(7):436–44.
54. Shadgan B, Menon M, Sanders D, et al. Current thinking about acute compartment syndrome of the lower extremity. Can J Surg 2010;53(5):329–34.
55. Kearns SR, Daly AF, Sheehan K, et al. Oral vitamin C reduces the injury to skeletal muscle caused by compartment syndrome. J Bone Jt Surg Br Vol 2004;86-B(6): 906–11.
56. Better OS, Zinman C, Reis DN, et al. Hypertonic mannitol ameliorates intracompartmental tamponade in model compartment syndrome in the dog. NEF 1991; 58(3):344–6.
57. Odland R, Schmidt AH, Hunter B, et al. Use of tissue ultrafiltration for treatment of compartment syndrome: a pilot study using porcine hindlimbs. J Orthop Trauma 2005;19(4):267–75.

Moving?

Make sure your subscription moves with you!

To notify us of your new address, find your **Clinics Account Number** (located on your mailing label above your name), and contact customer service at:

Email: journalscustomerservice-usa@elsevier.com

800-654-2452 (subscribers in the U.S. & Canada)
314-447-8871 (subscribers outside of the U.S. & Canada)

Fax number: 314-447-8029

Elsevier Health Sciences Division
Subscription Customer Service
3251 Riverport Lane
Maryland Heights, MO 63043

*To ensure uninterrupted delivery of your subscription, please notify us at least 4 weeks in advance of move.